I0438100

ALL DIETS DIE

How to Win & Be Thin (for life!)

John L. Pantera

authorHOUSE®

AuthorHouse™
1663 Liberty Drive
Bloomington, IN 47403
www.authorhouse.com
Phone: 1-800-839-8640

First published by AuthorHouse 6/24/2009

ISBN: 978-1-4389-8188-8 (e)
ISBN: 978-1-4389-8186-4 (sc)
ISBN: 978-1-4389-8187-1 (hc)

Printed in the United States of America
Bloomington, Indiana
This book is printed on acid-free paper.

CONTENTS

SECTION III
The Ultimate Fat Burning Exercise Plan (Simplified)

MEDICAL DISCLAIMER

All information is intended for your general knowledge only and is not a substitute for medical advice or treatment for specific medical conditions. You should seek prompt medical care for any specific health issues and consult your physician before starting a new fitness or nutrition regimen.

The information contained in this book is presented in summary form only and intended to provide broad consumer understanding and knowledge of nutrition, exercise and dietary supplements. The information should not be considered complete and should not be used in place of a visit, call, consultation or advice of your doctor, specialist or other health care provider.

The author does not recommend the self-management of health problems. Information obtained by using this program does not cover all diseases, ailments, physical conditions, nor does it cover their subsequent treatment. Should you have any health care related questions, please call your doctor or other health care provider promptly. You should never disregard medical advice or delay in seeking it because of something you have read or hear.

The use of nutrition and exercise to lose weight and/or control metabolic disorders and disease is a very complicated process, and is not the purpose of this book. The sole purpose of this book is to help healthy people reach their personal fitness and wellness goals by educating them in proper nutrition and exercise basics.

The author is not a medical doctor, registered dietitian, or clinical nutritionist; the author is a fitness and nutrition coach and does not make any other professional claim.

Your personal nutrition plan will not be the answer all by itself. You must also exercise on a regular basis and maintain sound healthy habits, including regular visits to your doctor. No results or specific expectations are guaranteed whatsoever from following the guidelines in this book. If you have been sedentary and are unaccustomed to any level of exercise, you should obtain your doctor's clearance before beginning an exercise program.

The author and publisher shall have neither liability nor responsibility to any person or entity with respect to any of the information contained in this book. The reader assumes all risk for any injury, loss or damage caused or alleged to be caused, directly or indirectly by actions taken in response to the information provided in this program.

ABOUT THE AUTHOR

Allow me to introduce myself. My name is John L. Pantera. I am many things. First, let me tell you what I am not.

I am not a traditional wellness author, in that I do not claim to have the latest and greatest "new" diet program that will miraculously melt away body fat with little or no effort. I am not a believer in magic pills or gimmicks that you've most likely seen on late night television. I also am not under any pressure whatsoever from any source of media that might influence the content of what you are about to read, which means that you now have access to a non-biased, simplified and proven lifestyle program that does not offer any empty promises, period.

I realize that by taking a non-traditional approach I am unlikely to produce a bestseller. That's okay with me. I'm not doing this for the money. I'm not doing this for fame. I am doing this for the regular, everyday person out there that is lost in their personal journey to a healthy lifestyle, and maybe needs some help. Most of us are confused when it comes to losing body fat and staying fit and lean for good. My goal is to eliminate that confusion.

Now, on to what I am. I am a regular everyday person. I enjoy the simple things in life. I am a family man. I love and respect others and myself. I am passionate about fitness and nutrition, and changing people's lives. I have a deep passionate affection for food, especially greasy, salty dishes. Let's not forget my own personal love for chocolate. Sound familiar?

You see, we are all the same to a certain degree. We all have pleasures, desires, temptations and weaknesses. The bad news is for most of us these vices often apply directly to food and weight gain. The great news is that I have simplified the fat loss process and weeded through all of the useful (and use-less) information floating around out there regarding healthy living and weight loss. The result is this book, which is the last ~~diet~~ *lifestyle* book you will ever need (no more use of the word diet).

Some more about what I am: I am a Body Transformation Expert. I help people change their lives and transform their bodies through nutrition, exercise and wellness. I am a Specialist in Performance Nutrition (SPN) as well as a Certified Fitness Trainer (CFT) through the International Sports Sciences Association (ISSA), a well-respected leader in the health and wellness industry. Virtually all of my clients are between the ages of 34-65, with some exceptions, and most of them desperately need to lose body fat, get healthy and return to the way they used to look and feel. See, I deal with regular people. I don't typically deal with athletes or people that are already successful on their own. This program does apply to everyone that wishes to be super lean and fit, regardless of their current fitness level, but it is directly targeted at the ordinary adult who needs help.

I have been coaching and transforming my clients through nutrition planning and exercise for well over ten years, and have contributed to hundreds of amazing success stories. I also consider myself to be a firm believer in what I preach, and not only do I use the principles in this book to transform my clients, I practice them as well.

I am hoping that my credentials and personal mantras are sufficient enough to convince you that the information in this book is worth your while. I have chosen a format for this book that is in plain English so that it is easy to read, simple to understand and, most importantly, applies to your situation. You will not find a lot of scientific jargon and confusing principles, just simple steps in layman's terms so that you fully understand how to transform your body for life. It's also my hope that you'll be able to explain it to others. Heaven knows that our younger generation certainly needs some unbiased guidance in losing body fat, so my goal is to educate both you and your family in this quest for health.

There are a few things to note about this book and its contents: (1) this program is not a gimmick. In fact, most of what you read you will find you already know or knew at some point in time, (2) everything in this book focuses on improving your health from a long-term lifestyle perspective, not an overnight quick fix (you know those don't work), and (3) all of the information contained in this book is results-driven and proven, and while there is plenty of science behind the principles, I have limited the amount of specific references in order to keep the fat loss process simple. Simple terms work best in my world, and you will be surprised at just how much of this information you will retain after starting this program. It really is simple.

Lastly, I dedicate this book to anyone who has ever struggled to achieve a goal. There is nothing quite like overcoming adversity. Anyone that has ever reached a significant goal will tell you that without resistance, there is no success. Losing body fat and choosing a fit and healthy lifestyle is one of the most difficult roads to take. You have found this book one way or another, or maybe it found you. Whatever the case, it happened for a reason. And as it turns out, it's dedicated to YOU!

INTRODUCTION

First of all, congratulations! This is it, the moment you've been waiting for...no more sifting through countless articles and books trying to find out what is real and what is designed to sell as the "newest breakthrough in losing body fat." No more New Year's resolutions. No more feeling guilty about food, no more ups and downs and yo-yo dieting. The time has come, and it is NOW.

We will start at the most important and critical principles of them all: setting goals and positive affirmations. I will guide you through the reasons why **all diets die** and explain the roots of the obesity problem that many Americans face today. I'll also fill you in on how to avoid that trap.

You will learn all about the secrets of losing body fat and the difference between body fat and body weight. We will cover the basics of your metabolism as well as how to properly balance your meals to ignite the metabolic flame you have inside of you! You will be the expert on losing body fat the correct way without the empty promises, and best of all, your fat loss success will be permanent.

I will teach you about the role of water in your success, as well as discuss the truth behind the supplement industry; there are a lot of misconceptions regarding which supplements you should use and which ones you should avoid at all costs.

Exercise will not be ignored. I will simplify the myths and misconceptions of exercising and make sure that you are confident in knowing exactly what needs to be done to maximize your body fat loss success.

I need to be honest with you, just like I am with all of my

clients: this will take some work. It will not be easy. The principles and knowledge that you will gain from this book will be easy to understand, that I promise. What you do with this information is the hard part. We'll get there together; I am committed to helping you.

You've taken the first step, which is to make a change in your life. The hardest part is now behind you. Don't worry I'll be with you every step the way. Now let's get started!

SECTION I

WHERE DO I BEGIN?

CHAPTER 1:

Americans Are Getting Fatter Each Year: Why all diets die and ultimately cause you to fail

"Let us eat and drink, for tomorrow we diet."
- Wendy Morgan

"Enjoy life. Think of all the women who passed up dessert on the Titanic."
- Unknown

"In general, mankind, since the improvement of cookery, eat about twice as much as nature requires."
- Benjamin Franklin

Okay, let's get it out there: Americans are in trouble! As a nation, we have never been collectively more overweight than we are now. I'm sure you've heard that before, and with all of our technological advances and so much information at our fingertips, it's sometimes shocking that we haven't all figured out the big fat loss mystery.... right?

There are several reasons for this weight gain phenomenon, and depending on who you talk to, you'll get more than one viewpoint. The most obvious factors are the following:

1. As a whole, Americans have drastically reduced the amount of calories we burn throughout the day. This is

due to our society moving from an extremely laborious workplace to much more of a technological workplace, where most of us work sitting at a desk. Even our children have become virtually inactive, with a drop in gym class requirements and a rise in video game popularity.

2. The amount of processed food we ingest has increased tenfold, diminishing the amount of macro and micronutrients that come from natural sources of food.

3. Because we are all in a rush, we seek convenience when we eat, which usually leads us to fast food spots and large portions on the go. Or even worse, we neglect or even forget to eat altogether, causing a massive metabolic slowdown. Also, most of us eat out quite often, and the portion sizes here in America are HUGE! The average size of a dinner out is a big enough portion to feed 3 adults. Yet most of us clean our plate each and every time we dine out, not to mention the double portion of wine or the 22oz. draft beer, dessert and coffee specialty drinks.

4. We all have tried different fad diets, and without question, the fad diet ended abruptly, or died. In the process, most of us have triggered a starvation response in our bodies due to the low-calorie nature of most diets. We will talk later about your metabolism, but this process of starving yourself and subsequently 'falling off the wagon' causes a drastic change in the way our bodies digest and process calories. Many ups and downs of this pattern that cause us to repeatedly gain and lose weight, or the "yo-yo effect," greatly contribute to our inability to correctly and permanently lose body fat.

5. There is an overwhelming amount of information on losing body fat, including diet books, exercise programs, and infomercials promising 5-minute solutions – this is because the weight loss industry is a multi-billion dollar industry. Clearly, the demand is being exploited for profit. Every month there seems to be a new breakthrough program or pill or machine that has never been discovered

until now! Many of us jump on the bandwagon hoping that our body fat woes will disappear with little or no effort. So, without changing our lifestyles, we are falling into that yo-yo pattern yet again, and none of us seem to know what path to take for permanent results.

6. Drugs, medications, diet pills and other unnatural substances have done a number on our bodies through the years. Too many of us have surrendered to popping pills for "health" rather than getting back to the basics of sound nutrition and exercise. These unnatural substances have severe effects on our digestive, endocrine, circulatory and central nervous systems, not to mention the fact that they contribute significantly to weight gain.

These are just some of the factors; there are many more. The bottom line is that you now have a choice. You are at a crossroads. Path #1 is the path you have been on up until now. If you had stayed on that path, it would continue to lead you on a frustrating roller coaster of up and down weight gain/loss. Path #2 is the path of truth. The instant you began reading this book, you veered off Path #1 and began down the path of truth. Way to go!

FACT: ALL DIETS DIE!

The definition of a diet, according to the Merriam-Webster dictionary, is the following: **diet;** *a regimen of eating and drinking sparingly so as to reduce one's weight.* This has always been interesting to me, and if you read it twice you'll notice a couple of things. First, the word *sparingly* is used. This implies a low calorie regimen. With a low calorie regimen comes the feeling of deprivation and restriction. This hardly sounds like a lifestyle change, and very difficult to maintain long-term.

Secondly, the goal is just to reduce one's *weight* – not fat. We will discuss the difference between body weight and body fat later, so keep this in mind. All diets work to some degree if losing *weight* is your only goal. If you want to permanently lose *body fat*, this definition is not the answer.

Lastly, it says nothing about maintaining a long-term result or permanent change. This implies that a diet is temporary until the goal is met. Most of us have seen some success from a diet, but once the diet dies, we gain the weight back and then some. This is the most frustrating and damaging part of the dieting cycle.

Dieting has been around for quite some time. The concept of the diet gained popularity throughout the 1980's with the emergence of countless fad diets; it'll make your head spin if you take a look back to that time. Do you remember the cabbage soup diet? How about the grapefruit diet? Then along came the diet revolution that was headlined by the Atkins diet, the Zone diet and more recently the South Beach diet.

While many of these fad diets of the past certainly had good intentions, they are all seriously flawed, and some downright unhealthy. I will not point fingers or single out any one diet mentioned above. Rather, let's look at some reasons why many diets, such as these, ultimately fail (and eventually die), causing you to feel and look worse off than when you began.

THE HUMAN BODY'S NATURAL STARVATION TRIGGERS

The human body is a wonderful and beautiful thing. We are alive! Our bodies, regardless of your belief system, have evolved over many centuries to adapt to our physical and mental needs in order to promote survival. Throughout the years, as humans went from being hunters and gatherers to a more agricultural/industrial society, our process of eating food and drinking fluids has changed dramatically. We now know where our next meal will come from, and we have so many choices to fulfill that task. Food processing and distribution is big business in this day and age, especially here in America.

Long ago, we did not have such a luxury. Families had to rely on their own ability to hunt for food and sometimes went weeks if not months without nourishment. For that reason, the human body took on certain metabolic functions in order to slow down the rate at which calories are burned in order to allow for long periods of "starvation." The good news from this is that we can actually live without food for many weeks. The bad news is that we no longer need this natural benefit, and this survival mechanism has now been working against us while we attempt to lose body fat. Let me explain…

A typical adult female, let's call her Jane, decides to start a diet. Jane has tried all the diets. Over the years she had gained and lost the same 50 pounds multiple times. With every diet she began, she saw great results, typically losing a quick 15 pounds. After a few weeks, the weight loss started to fizzle, and when she did her twice-daily weigh in on her scale, it just seemed to stop moving. Before long, she gained all of her weight back, and a few extra pounds to boot. Sound familiar?

Here's the problem. This is undoubtedly the most damaging cycle a human being can put their body through, and it seems as though most of us at some point have followed this pattern. It starts with a very low calorie diet. As with most diets, low calories leads to an initial weight loss, most of that weight being water weight. Because we see a drop on the scale, we keep going and think that we are actually succeeding.

Very quickly, our bodies catch on to the fact that we are slowly depriving ourselves of key nutrients and enough calories to sustain our muscle mass and give us energy. Because the body does not know where the next meal is coming from (the hunter/gatherer defense mechanism), the body is smart enough to slow down the rate at which we absorb, digest and use calories. This is your metabolism! And it is slowing down!

What happens next is that our system gets used to a lower rate, and when we do actually eat food, that food gets processed very slowly. It's important to note that your metabolism declines with age naturally, something we cannot change. But what we are doing in this cycle is pushing along the natural aging process so that our bodies are acting as if we are much older than we really are. Does that sound like it's a good thing?

The worst part is when the diet stops. Inevitably we go off the diet, because no one can restrict the foods they love forever, nor should anyone have to. So, our calorie total for the day shoots way back up. Guess what? Our metabolism is so slow that our body simply cannot process the excess calories and those extra calories end up getting stored away as body fat! Anyone that has ever been a victim of this knows that feeling. The weight seems to go back on about ten times faster than it went away. Not fun!

Too many of us repeat this viscous cycle for years and years, and each time our internal systems grow weaker and slower. Obviously this is frustrating, and when the weight comes back you feel like a failure. So we give up completely.

THERE IS SO MUCH MISLEADING INFORMATION OUT THERE!

Go to Google.com and search the word "diet." There are over 26,000,000 results that pop up! I think it's safe to say that diets are a popular thing, and that most adults have tried at least one diet at some point in their life. There certainly is no shortage of information on the topic, and the truth of the matter is that over 90% of the information you find out there on dieting is misleading, false or downright unhealthy.

How can this be? One word: GREED. There have been, and continue to be, countless ways for individuals and companies to make a lot of money selling diet pills, drinks, exercise gimmicks and the newest, greatest fad that can be thought up. As a result of the rapidly growing fat loss market, a wave of bad information has flooded the Internet and the book stores, resulting in more confusion than ever.

Are carbs good or bad? Should I limit my fat intake, or is high protein the way to go? Does the the Ab Wheel really work that well? What's all the fuss about the Atkins Diet? Is the South Beach Diet better? How about cleansing? There's a diet pill now endorsed by the FDA, so it must work, right? Phew...that's a lot of options, and a lot of different opinions. Most of my clients have expressed much confusion and the feeling of being overwhelmed each year with the newest fad weight loss gimmick.

While dieting through the years and gaining and losing weight, people have done so in often unhealthy ways due to the misconceptions of exactly how to do it right. This ongoing cycle has caused most Americans, adults and children alike, to be severely overweight and unhealthy, and trends seem to be getting worse.

THE CYCLE ENDS NOW

There is hope. I can tell you first hand that many people that I have worked with have been through the yo-yo and the roller coaster for years upon years only to ultimately give up on their situation… until they decided to do it right.

In order to break this cycle and to look and feel the way you want to, you must commit to change! You must commit to give up on all gimmicks and diets, and commit to changing your lifestyle. Presented to you in this book is all of the tools and knowledge you will need to dispel any myths and cut a crystal clear path to success. If you can't commit, stop reading now and give this book to someone else. If you CAN, keep reading – your life is about to change for **GOOD**!

RAPID RECAP

1. There are many significant reasons why most Americans are obese in these days and times. Despite what your struggle might be, there is a way out.

2. The word "diet" implies temporary results and losing weight, not body fat. All diets eventually die.

3. Your body has a natural way of surviving when faced with a severe calorie restriction. This "starvation response" happens when you diet for too long, and it causes your

metabolism to slow down. This makes it virtually impossible to lose body fat.

4. There is so much bad information out there it is no wonder people are confused. Most of the information presented to you is misleading and unhealthy. You will now learn the true way to be healthy and lean for life.

CHAPTER 2:

Where to Start: The power of the positive mind and effective (yet easy) goal setting

"Always bear in mind that your own resolution to succeed is more important than any one thing."
- Abraham Lincoln

Stephen R. Covey said it best in his book The 7 Habits of Highly Effective People: Begin with the end in mind. You've heard it many times before, and it's become somewhat of a cliché these days, but how can you get to where you're going without knowing where you want to be? Too often people neglect to set goals in their personal and professional lives, and guess what happens? They end up not getting there.

Also, too many clients in the past that I have seen had the wrong perspective on their situation, and I witnessed many self-fulfilling prophecies of failure. Henry Ford had one of the all-time classic motivational quotes when he said, "Whether you think you can or you can't, either way you're right."

This chapter will focus on two things: positive affirmations and goal setting. I will simplify this for you so that it is easy yet very powerful. This might be the most important chapter in this book, because it's all about getting your head on straight to succeed! Without the right mindset and without a crystal clear roadmap of where you're going, nothing else matters.

WHY MOST PEOPLE NEVER ACHIEVE THEIR GOALS

Fact: 98% of people do not have written goals. I realize that you probably fit into that 98%, but the good news is that it's okay, that's why we're here! That ends today. When I think about why most of us do not write down our goals, a few reasons come to mind:

1. We discount the importance of writing down our goals.
2. We have no idea what we would like to accomplish.
3. We are afraid of failure.
4. We are afraid of success (yes, this does happen, I'll explain this one below...).
5. We don't have time (my all-time favorite excuse!).
6. We don't know how to put our goals into a format that makes sense.
7. We have no personal emotional reasons for achieving our goals.
8. We have no one to hold us accountable!
9. We haven't ever thought about setting goals ("the thought never entered into my mind").
10. We feel our goals are unattainable, so why bother?

Do any of these thoughts ever cross your mind when goal setting is mentioned? Don't worry, you're not alone. Most people fall into one or more of these categories, and it's very easy to think that goal setting is a waste of time. Sometimes we simply don't know what we want, or we are afraid that if we set a goal and don't make it we are failures. Some people are scared to reach their goal because that means they will now have to reach even higher. That's being afraid of success, and it is more common than you think. Whatever your reason for not writing down your goals might be, you are now required to take action and get this critical task done.

EVERYTHING YOU NEED TO GET STARTED NOW!

Let's make this process simple. You may have heard of the S.M.A.R.T.S. acronym that is often used to set goals and track them, and below you will find a form that utilizes that acronym, but with a slight twist. The S.M.A.R.T.S. acronym stands for *Specific*, *Measurable*, *As* if Now, *Recorded*, *Timeframe* and *Shared*. I have used this format of setting and tracking goals not only for myself throughout the years but with hundreds of clients that wanted to look and feel great and didn't know where to start. Let's quickly dive into each element of this acronym and then finally get your goals in ink.

First, we start with *Specific*. Too often someone will think of something they would like to accomplish and may even get as far as to write it down, but it turns out to be too vague or general. In this case, it is very difficult to tell whether or not the goal has been accomplished, or if it is even reasonable. The more specific the goal the better chances you will have at zeroing in on that goal. For example, if your goal is to lose weight, simply saying "I would like to lose weight" has no crystal clear end in mind. An improved version of this statement would be "I need to lose 15 pounds of body fat over the next 16 weeks." We will improve this even more as we go through this goal setting exercise, but you get the point. Our goals must be specific or we lose the ability to self-reflect on our success. Without specific goals, you simply cannot have a plan of action toward achieving results.

Next comes <u>*M*</u>easurable. This piece is critical and it goes in conjunction with <u>*S*</u>pecific. Without being able to measure your progress or whether or not a goal has been accomplished, how can you ever know where you stand? Again, avoid the trap of being too vague. Every goal must be measurable in order for you to be truly be satisfied with the outcome. Referring back to the previous example, setting a goal of losing weight is a good start, but how much weight do you intend to lose? Is it just weight or is it body fat? If your goal is to just lose weight, sit in a sauna for 30 minutes and weigh yourself, I guarantee a couple of water weight pounds will be shed and your goal is accomplished! Your goal must be measurable. Without this significant factor, you will wander aimlessly wondering if you've reached the pinnacle or not.

<u>*A*</u>s if Now is a bit different than most formats for tracking goals. Usually the 'A' stands for <u>*A*</u>ttainable, so bear with me as we go through this interesting yet powerful twist. The 'A' now stands for <u>*A*</u>s if Now, meaning that you will write out your goals in the present tense, as if you have already accomplished them. Your subconscious mind is a very powerful thing. What you truly believe (even if you have to lie to yourself) is what you will become. For this reason, you must write out your goals in the present tense as if the goal has already been achieved. For example, instead of "I would like to lose 20 pounds in 6 months," write it out to be "I have lost 20 pounds in 6 months and I look and feel great!" By assuming that you have already accomplished this goal, your subconscious mind will start to tell to you to act as if you are there already. And guess what happens? You start doing the things that you should be doing in order to bring you to that end result! A little skeptical? Don't worry, you're not alone. But I challenge you to truly give this a try, and see what happens. You may be pleasantly surprised.

<u>*R*</u>ecorded. This one is easy. You either write it down or you don't. <u>*R*</u>ecorded is pass/fail. An ancient Chinese proverb once stated that "goals that are not written down are merely wishes." How true this really is! It is so easy to say what you want to achieve, but it takes commitment to actually write it down in pen. Then it becomes real. Through this process, writing down your goals and "wishes"

formalizes your commitment.

*T*imeframe. You must have a specific timeline for each goal in order to create some urgency for yourself. If there is no timeline, there is no deadline! In the past I have broken out three tiers of timeframe with my clients: 90 days, 6 months and 1 year (or longer). It is important to have some short-term goals that don't seem to be too far away where they can be forgotten. It is also helpful to have a couple of long-term goals as well in order to help you see the big picture and work towards that end result. Without a timeframe, any of these goals, whether short- or long-term, are not likely to be a priority.

*S*hared. You must share your plans and dreams and goals with others that you care about and who care about you in return. If you don't, no one will be there to hold you accountable. Most people don't mind failing if they happen to be the only one that knows they failed. However, a person is much more likely to not want to fail if someone else knows their intentions. When setting your goals, share them with your spouse, significant other, family, friends, and anyone else that might be part of your support network. This final and critical step makes your goals real and unavoidable.

Now you have all of the tools and understanding to start setting your goals and begin achieving them. Below is a template for you to set your goals and get them in ink:

S-M-A-R-T-S GOALS

SMARTS = Specific-Measurable-As If Now-Attainable-Recorded-Timeframe-Shared

Name: ____________________ Date: ______

Mission: Write a set of goals that you are passionate about achieving. Below, write the emotional reasons why you must achieve these goals.

90 Day Goals

1.
2.
3.

6 Month Goals

1.
2.
3.

One Year + Goals

1.
2.
3.

**Emotional reasons why I must achieve these goals:

1.
2.
3.

<u>STOP HERE!!!</u> If you have just skipped the last page and said to yourself, "I'll do this part later" or "I don't really need this part," then close this book right now and give it to someone else that is serious about their fat loss plan. You cannot afford to skip the goal section; without that piece, nothing else I will teach you will mean anything! This is where it all starts. If you did complete the template, way to go! You are well on your way. If not, be honest with yourself and either take a few minutes and do it now or don't do it at all!

THE POWER OF THE POSITIVE MIND

Too often people will begin a diet or fat loss regimen with the ongoing thought running through their head that they will eventually fail. There is an old proverb that states, "We are what we think about all day long." If we think we will fail, we will. If we think we will always be fat, guess what? Our minds will bring us to that conclusion. The human mind is a very powerful thing, especially on a subconscious level. The subconscious mind does not know right or wrong or best intentions, it just directs our conscious mind to whatever we are thinking about.

I teach my clients to use positive affirmations to combat this ongoing cycle of negativity. Affirmations can be used in a number of ways to be constant reminders of what you are striving towards, and are very powerful when put to good use. Some examples include the following:

1. Keeping a daily journal to write down 3-5 positive affirmations each day. Remember, writing something down makes it permanent and more real.

2. Keeping Post-It notes with positive affirmations in strategic places, such as on the fridge or on the steering wheel of your car where they can't be ignored.

3. Using meditation and verbal repetition to reinforce the positive affirmations that will help you to stay on track.

4. Listening to self-improvement CD's or reading books

that support your goals. There certainly is no shortage of these types of media these days.

5. Using hypnotherapy to emphasize and strengthen your belief system in yourself and to assist in resisting weak points.

Below are some examples of positive affirmations that I have used and recommended to virtually all of my clients. Now remember, you must use these well before they are actually true. Your thoughts and beliefs will bring you to that end result. Do not wait until you've reached your goal to use the following affirmations, use them NOW:

- I am so grateful for my health and I continue to be in the best shape of my life.
- I fully deserve to be thin and healthy. I have worked so hard to get here.
- I have lost 20 pounds of body fat and look great!
- I am teaching my kids the importance of being healthy and eating right and I am leading by example.
- I am strong, I am healthy, and my life is great! I am so proud of how far I have come.
- I always reach my goals and hold myself accountable. If I can't, I seek the help of others.
- I now fit into those skinny jeans that have been in my closet for years.
- I make heads turn because I look and feel so great!
- My blood pressure is the lowest it has been in over 20 years!
- My doctor is amazed at how I was able to kick the cholesterol meds and get my numbers in check.

- I cannot wait for the next holiday or family get together so that I can shock everyone that thought I couldn't do it.

- Swimsuit season cannot come fast enough!

- I always eat well balanced meals and when I treat myself I feel no guilt because I have earned it.

- My spouse has been giving me those looks again. He/she can really tell that I have been working hard.

- I love to exercise. The feeling I get when I am done with my workout is unmatched!

- New challenges never intimidate me, I love stepping out of my comfort zone to try new things.

- I will never diet again. I have changed my lifestyle for good.

- By my next birthday, people I haven't seen will not recognize me.

- My metabolism is fast and high, constantly burning the calories I take in and using my body fat for fuel.

- My mirror is now my best friend, no longer my worst enemy!

These affirmations are very specific and they all assume that you are already there. But, they are only as good as how often you use them. It takes 21 days to form a habit, but 90 days to create permanent change.

My challenge to you is to write down some of these affirmations for 90 days straight. Before you know it, your attitude and your outlook will have changed, and you'll look forward to writing these down because you will be achieving them.

Below is a template to start writing down your daily positive affirmations today. No excuses, you've been given all of the tools... DO NOT skip this part of the program!!!!

MY DAILY POSITIVE AFFIRMATIONS

Rules: (1) Must be personal, use "I" and 'me", and start by stating "I am" or "I have", (2) must be in the present tense, and (3) must be positive!

Monday:
1.
2.
3.
Tuesday:
1.
2.
3.
Wednesday:
1.
2.
3.
Thursday:
1.
2.
3.
Friday:
1.
2.
3.
Saturday:
1.
2.
3.
Sunday:
1.
2.
3.

SUMMARY (SO FAR...)

Congratulations! The hardest part of this lifestyle change is over...you've got goals! You are armed with the most powerful weapon in history: your mind! You've just accomplished the **WHY** portion of your lifestyle change to come. Your goals and affirmations clearly outline why it is important for you to do this, and to do it right for the last time. No more temporary results. The next chapters in this book are all about the **HOW**. It won't be easy, but you can do it, I know you can. Let's get started.

RAPID RECAP

1. Goals are your roadmap to success. Unwritten goals are simply wishes that most likely won't come true.
2. Most people don't write down their goals. Be the minority.
3. Set 90 day, 6 month and long term goals so that you always have a target in your sights.
4. Use positive affirmations to become mentally strong and confident. Your mind is your most powerful muscle.

CHAPTER 3:

Accountability: Why each of us desperately needs it to succeed

"When a man points a finger at someone else, he should remember that four of his fingers are pointing at himself." – Louis Nizer

The definition of the word "accountability," according to Merriam-Webster's dictionary is "an obligation or willingness to accept responsibility or to account for one's actions."

Most of us at one point or another have had someone hold us accountable, even if we were unwilling at the time to be open to the idea. An example would be a high school coach or a teacher that always seemed to demand the best of us. At the time, you may have despised that person. We all have bad memories of that special someone telling you much of what you didn't want to hear, especially during the tough times. Yet, as you look back now, I'm willing to bet that person is pretty high up on your respect list.

That is the essence of true accountability, and without anyone to hold you accountable for your goals and actions, your likelihood of holding yourself accountable is very slim. Very few people in this world have the ability to be so self-disciplined, most notably with nutrition and exercise. The bottom line is, it's TOUGH! Even the world's best athletes have coaches and peers that hold them accountable.

There are many different places to find an accountability source. Let's start with self-accountability. In order to succeed at your fat loss goal, you must have some self-discipline and accountability to your goals. Make no mistake, this is the one thing that keeps people from succeeding in fat loss and any other goal they have. That is because self accountability is very difficult to do. We all have convincingly lied to ourselves at some point that we were going to change our lifestyle: "This will be my last diet..." Sound familiar?

WHAT MOTIVATES YOU?

In order to effectively hold yourself accountable, there must be a consequence to your actions. Some of us are motivated by positive reinforcement. If you do something, you earn or win a prize. Some, on the other hand, are pushed by negative reinforcement, or punishment. It's called the carrot and the stick principle. The first part of self-discipline is determining what motivates you, positive or negative. There is no right or wrong here, so you must be honest with yourself. Next, you must develop a reward/punishment system for yourself based on what motivates you.

If you are encouraged by positive reinforcement, then you must treat yourself when you have earned it. Here's the catch: you MUST truly earn your treat, and you MUST enjoy that treat without any guilt whatsoever! Otherwise, if you reward yourself and then feel bad about doing so, you risk falling back into the downward spiral of guilt and self-loathing which can derail you very quickly. The mental stresses that can be caused by feelings of guilt do more damage to you physically and mentally than the actual indulgence.

An example of how to reward yourself for doing well or reaching a goal is to set up a day of the week to enjoy your favorite indulgence. Let's say you love pizza. Who doesn't, right? So, if you have set a goal for the week to work out at least three times for forty-five minutes and stick to your nutrition plan from Monday through Friday, then plan on enjoying a pizza on Saturday night with a glass of wine and don't think twice about it! If you've truly done your best and worked hard, you deserve it! This method allows you to look forward to your special night as well as erase any bad feelings you may have towards your favorite foods.

If you happen to be pushed more by negative reinforcement (and don't worry, you're not alone!), then you must sacrifice something that is special to you if you allow yourself to fail. In order to effectively hold yourself accountable, there must be a consequence!

For instance, if you really can't stand the idea of doing cardiovascular workouts, then use that activity as your punishment for letting yourself down. If you slip up and overeat, then thirty minutes on the treadmill is your punishment. Or another example might be forfeiting your favorite weekly TV show as a correction to a poor behavior. It must be either something you have to give up that you love or something that will benefit you but you still don't enjoy. If the correction or punishment does not evoke an emotional response from you, then you are not catering to your style of reinforcement. It almost has to hurt a bit!

The next place to find an accountability source is from a friend or family member. This can be a great and effective place to seek out some accountability, but it can be tricky as well. In an ideal situation, the accountability source would be a neutral third-party that has no bias towards you. Oftentimes someone will pair up with a friend to lose weight and the two end up enabling each other to fall off the wagon. Or that friend doesn't want to hurt your feelings, so they back off when you are slipping. If you've paired up with a family member for accountability, they may feel awkward about the accountability relationship because holding someone accountable to a goal is not simple or easy. If you have someone in your circle or friends or family that can be unbiased, by all means use that person to help you.

However, it can work. I've seen it work. If you are going to ask for help from a friend or family member, the best way to stick to the plan is to have a contract. Not a verbal contract; that's too weak. What you will need is a rock-solid written contract stating the goals and purposes of linking up with each other in accountability, and some ramifications if one of the partners falls short of their duties.

You can make this contract as simple or complex as needed; just make sure you each have a copy. Put it somewhere that you can see it regularly.

Below is a sample of a contract I've used with clients in the past that clearly states the clients' goals as well as the specific accountability measures they are seeking from me. Feel free to use or modify this template; it is a powerful thing to get this agreement in writing. You are much more likely to break a verbal contract than you are a written one.

ACCOUNTABILITY CONTRACT

Name:

Accountability Partner:

Goal(s):

Why I Need Help:

If I am slipping, I give you permission to do the following:

If I fail or quit, I agree to give up the following (negative reinforcement):

When I succeed, I get to do or have the following (positive reinforcement):

____________________________ ____________________________

Signature #1 & date Signature #2 & date

If you are having trouble holding yourself accountable and staying disciplined, and your family or friends are not quite up to the task, then the third and final tactic to seek out an honest, non-biased source of responsibility is to hire a fitness trainer, nutritionist/dietician or some other coaching professional. As a Certified Fitness Trainer and Specialist in Performance Nutrition, accountability was the essence of my relationship with my clients. I truly loved to hold people accountable and every single time the client thanked me for it in the end. Believe me, it wasn't always easy, but my motto, which my clients quickly learned was true, was "hate me now, love me later."

Great trainers and coaches know that the end result is all that matters. A coach that will bring you to your goal is not trying to win a popularity contest. Of course, like any industry, there are great trainers and coaches and there are not so great ones as well. Here are some tips on deciding which professionals to use (and which ones to avoid!):

1. Only commit to someone that commits to you. Mutual accountability is a must!

2. When you first meet a potential coach, does he/she ask questions, or just tell you how they can help? Seek those that ask questions and get to the root of your struggles.

3. What licenses/certifications does this person have? Do your research on their resume.

4. Make sure your new coach matches your personality type; if you don't have fun in the process it won't last.

5. Look for honest expectations that are realistic. If someone sells you the "pie in the sky," don't fall for it. Make sure your coach sets goals with you that are measurable.

6. Check the environment where you will meet (gym, private studio, office, etc.) and make sure you are comfortable there.

7. Prevent yourself from quitting. Pay up front, that way you are responsible if you quit!

No matter which route you choose for accountability, seeking out help from others will always increase your success rate tenfold!

THE STORY OF PETER

One story I will share with you about accountability is the story of Peter. When I first started helping others transform their bodies, Peter was one of my first clients. He was in rough shape. Peter was a chain smoker for many years. At the time he was about forty pounds overweight and had several medications just to keep his blood pressure and cholesterol in check. On top of that, Peter's confidence level in himself and me was in the dumps. He was in desperate need of change, but he admitted to me immediately that he was his own worst enemy, and he was notorious for attempting to change on his own before eventually falling off of the wagon...hard!

Now, at that point in my career I hadn't really held anyone accountable to the extent that Peter needed me to. I was nervous, just as Peter was to get started. I honestly didn't even know where to begin. That's when I decided that we needed something in writing that would allow me to hold him accountable and prove to be a good reminder of why he wanted to change in the first place. I also needed to him to know that I was just as serious about his success as he was. So, we started with the same exact accountability contract that has been provided to you above.

From that simple one page document, everything changed. I would pull that document out at least twice a week when Peter would slip up or have a poor attitude. If he had a bad day and didn't feel like working out, that contract suddenly appeared in front of his face! He couldn't escape what he had agreed to, and I never let him lose sight of that. Likewise, if I was feeling off or if I had a bad day, I allowed Peter to tell it to me straight and remind me of why we were working together. Accountability is always a two-way street!

Again, I often used my favorite motto as a coach and trainer, "Hate me now, love me later," and believe me Peter surely had days when he hated me! The beginning of our relationship as client/

coach began back in 2003, and now Peter maintains a low body fat percentage, is stronger and healthier than he has ever been, and he's 59 years old! We still hold each other accountable on many things, but it all started with a simple agreement in writing to do so.

RAPID RECAP

1. Every one of us needs accountability to succeed at losing body fat. It is not easy, and it's near impossible to do on your own.

2. There are numerous sources of accountability you may seek. The hardest part is getting started and asking someone to help.

3. Find out what motivates you and use that to your advantage. Some are motivated by the positive, others by the negative. There is no right or wrong, only what will work best for you.

4. Use an accountability contract to solidify your commitment. Make your goals crystal clear and allow someone to tell you what you need to hear.

5. Great coaches and fitness professionals are often the best accountability sources because they are unbiased and well-trained in helping others lose body fat.

SECTION II

EVERYTHING YOU NEED TO KNOW ABOUT LOSING BODY FAT

CHAPTER 4:

The Concrete Laws of Losing Body Fat

"Preserving health by too severe a rule is a wearisome malady."
–La Rochefoucauld

"I burned sixty calories.
That should take care of a peanut I had in 1962."
- Rita Rudner

Losing body fat is a multi-billion dollar industry each year. There are literally thousands upon thousands of diet pills, exercise gimmicks and quick fixes that promise results or YOUR MONEY BACK!!! GAURANTEED!!! In this age of readily available information, one would think that the consumers would wise up to these infomercials. But we keep falling for them. With all of the awareness we now have towards wellness, coupled with our own mistakes of the past, how can we continue to deny the simple truths of how to lose body fat the correct (and permanent) way?

Well, that cycle ends here. In this chapter, I will teach you the five concrete laws of losing body fat. No more lies, no more gimmicks. This chapter will lay it all out for you in simple terms that cannot be negotiated. The following principles apply to everyone on this earth that wishes to lose unsightly and unhealthy body fat permanently.

LAW #1 - THE LAW OF THE CALORIE DEFICIT/SURPLUS

This law is simple. Yet so many people don't understand it, because while being simple in theory, most people don't really understand what a calorie is. What is a calorie? The easiest definition I can give you of a calorie is that it is a "measure of food (energy)." Calories help you to measure how much food you eat and how much energy your body needs on a daily basis. You do not need to know the scientific breakdown of how or why calories came about as a means of measuring our food, so let's keep it simple.

When you are ingesting food, no matter what food it is, the nutrients of that food can be broken down into three broad categories or macronutrients. The three macronutrients of food are (1) protein, (2) carbohydrates and (3) fats. Each of these macronutrients has a caloric value attached to it. For example, one gram of protein is equal to four calories. The same goes for carbohydrates, which are equal to four calories per gram. However, one gram of fat equals nine calories.

In any given day, your body requires a certain number of total calories in order to maintain healthy function, proper bone mass and muscle mass. Your body also is looking for a regular balance of where your calories come from, or macronutrient balance. That means of your total daily calories, a certain amount should come from protein, some from carbs, and some from healthy fats. Your total number of daily calories and your specific nutrient balance will be unique to you, we will discuss that further in just a bit.

So we know that calories are a way to measure your nutrients from your food. With that information, we can now learn Law #1:

<u>The Law of the Calorie Deficit/Surplus</u> – *If you eat fewer calories per day than your daily amount required to maintain your current weight, you will lose weight (calorie deficit). If you eat more calories per day than your daily amount required to maintain your current weight, you will gain weight (calorie surplus).*

This law does not bend or waiver; it is concrete. This is the one law that can trump all other weight loss and diet strategies. If your plan is to lose body fat, you must follow this simple rule.

When your body is in a calorie deficit (fewer calories than your body needs to maintain your current weight) then stored body fat will be tapped into as a fuel source, and you will lose weight. This is because you are not providing your body with the nutrients it wants, so your body seeks out those nutrients elsewhere. One place it looks: your stored body fat.

When your body is in a calorie surplus (more calories than your body needs to maintain your current weight) then those extra calories will get stored away as body fat.

This seems prretty simple, right? There is a catch…

LAW #2 – THE LAW OF PORTIONS

If you were born and raised in America, than you know full well that we Americans do everything to the fullest, especially eating and drinking! Portion control in this country is a punch line these days, and many people are in the overweight state they are in due to a lack of portion control. I'll be the first to admit it, eating is fun! Eating is comforting! When you are eating something you truly love, it is hard to stop. And of course, most foods that we love happen to be high in calories as well, so it's a double whammy!

Taking Law #1 and expanding on it, we come to the Law of Portions:

<u>The Law of Portions</u> – *even if you are in a calorie deficit for the day, if you have too many calories at one sitting, the body can only process so many calories at once and the excess calories will be stored as body fat. You must spread your total calories throughout the day into smaller, portion-controlled meals.*

This is where most people, me included, really struggle. Oftentimes we have a bad day and take out our frustrations on a gallon of ice cream. I've been there; you are not alone. Or, we go out to dinner and the portions put in front of us are enormous, and of course we don't want to be rude so we clean our plate. Abiding by this law is not easy. In fact, it's downright hard. But in order to truly succeed at your fat loss goal, you mustn't sabotage your hard work by binge eating. Lack of portion control can erase a day's worth of discipline in just a few short minutes.

So, how do you maintain good portion control? Here are some tips on how to win at the battle of portions:

1. When you go out to eat, have your waiter or waitress bring you your meal cut in half, with the other half packed up to-go. Most restaurants will cater to this request – all you need to do is ask.

2. When cooking for yourself or for your family, pull out the Tupperware before you sit down to eat. This will remind you that a portion of what you just cooked must be packed away for tomorrow's lunch.

3. Don't feel the need to clean your plate. As children we are taught that it is bad to not finish all of your food, even if it means overeating after feeling full. Leftovers should be a staple in your house.

4. Eat fibrous foods with every meal. Fiber curbs your hunger and makes you feel full. For example, enjoy a mixed greens salad with plenty of vegetables before your meal. You will find that you will not be able to have such big portions, you will already feel satisfied!

5. Drink plenty of water. We will discuss the role of water in a later chapter, but please know that water can also satisfy major hunger pangs that you may experience. Drink 16oz. of water prior to a meal.

6. By spreading out meals/snacks into 5-6 occurrences per day, you will fell much less hungry when it comes to dinner time. More frequent meals means less portions per meal.

7. Be accountable! Hold yourself accountable, have your spouse or coach hold you accountable, and/or hold your children accountable. You must practice what you preach!

LAW #3 – THE LAW OF ACTIVITY (YOU NEED TO MOVE!!!)

All too often people will start a diet with the thinking that they need to restrict calories and just let the fat starve off. "If I cut my calories enough, I will lose this weight." Have you ever had that mentality? It's okay, most of us have at one point. We find ourselves literally starving ourselves, hoping that the excess body fat will disappear and never come back. 99% of diets that exists today preach a severe restriction on our daily caloric intake. And why not? That is the easy way to do it! You don't need to work hard, you don't need to exercise, you just need to restrict. No problem! Right?

Wrong! If you have ever tried to cut your calories to lose weight, you know just how hard it can get, and how little fun it can be. Ever been to a party and not been able to enjoy the food? That's not fun or easy. Ever been so hungry while on a diet that you felt sick to your stomach and run down? Again, not so fun, not so easy. I am here to tell you that any diet or lifestyle plan that preaches calorie cutting is severely flawed. I am also here to tell you to EAT!

Doesn't that sound like fun? Eating should be enjoyable and should be cherished. It should be social and communal and never looked upon as being bad. The fact is this: your body needs calories and nutrients not only to live, but to move, breath, talk, think, smile, and function! Cutting calories has many detriments, including a decrease in energy, muscle mass, health function, metabolism, brain activity and sex drive. So, to sum up the typical diet, you successfully become lethargic, weak, unhealthy, slower, dumber and you lose your libido!

Rather than starve off the stored body fat, you must learn to consistently burn off stored body fat by engaging in activity.

<u>The Law of Activity</u> – *starving off excess body fat (i.e. the typical diet known today) in simply unacceptable. In order to lose body fat permanently and maintain health and a high metabolism, you must eat enough calories to sustain your body, and actively burn off any excess fat through exercise.*

The most important factor that is behind this law is your metabolism. When cutting calories, your body turns to what is known as "starvation mode." We talked about this principle earlier. It's your body's way of surviving since it doesn't know where your next meal is coming from. Your metabolism slows down naturally as you age, and by restricting your calories you are decreasing your metabolic rate even further and causing most of the food that you ingest to be stored away for survival.

I will discuss what level of calories you will need each day in just a bit. For now, just know this: cutting calories is not the answer. You may lose weight in the beginning, but I assure you the weight you lose is mostly water weight and muscle mass, not body fat! Most people see the scale move down during the initial phases of a new diet and think that it is working. This could not be any further from the real truth. Your new mindset should involve a commitment to never sacrificing your metabolism. You will eat the right foods and the right amount of those foods so that you will never feel starved again. And, instead of starving off your body fat, you will burn it off.

A simple guideline as to how much activity is needed is to aim for 30-60 minutes of exercise 3-5 times per week. There is no right or wrong when it comes to movement and exercise. In later chapters I will outline an exercise program that is simple yet very effective at helping to burn off stored body fat calories.

LAW #4 – THE LAW OF CUSTOMIZATION

Any diet that claims to work for everyone will fail for most. We are all unique people, not only with respect to our personalities and our quirks, but also with respect to our bodies. We all require different amounts of exercise and calories, and we all have different lifestyles and commitments that will allow us to make the necessary changes to succeed. Some factors that help to determine what will work for you include your age, your body fat loss goal, your previous successes and failures, your support network around you and your ability to dedicate time.

The Law of Customization – *cookie cutter diets and exercise plans will not work for everyone. We all have specific needs. In order to find what works for you, you must use both calculation and gut instinct. Only through trial and error will one fully know what works for them, as well as what doesn't.*

We will use the law of customization for two reasons: (1) to determine how many calories you need on a daily basis to reach your goal, and (2) to be mindful that your exercise plan must be something you enjoy and have time to dedicate to, otherwise you will quit.

DETERMINING YOUR CALORIC NEEDS – THE KATCH-MCARDLE FORMULA

According to the American College of Sports Medicine (ACSM), which is one the leading authorities on losing body fat correctly, the lowest amount of calories an adult woman should ever take in per day is 1,200, and for an adult man that number is 1,800. I repeat: the LOWEST amount of calories per day. Many diets and programs today preach calorie levels much lower than that, which we now know causes the starvation response and slows down the metabolism.

Your daily caloric needs depend on several factors. According to the renowned physiologists Frank Katch and William McArdle, one's daily caloric needs can be calculated using a simple two-step formula that includes the most important factors of customization: your body fat percentage and your activity level. The first step of the formula is as follows:

Basal Metabolic Rate (BMR) = 370 + (21.6 X Lean Body Mass in kg)

This first step calculates what is known as your Basal Metabolic Rate, or BMR. Your BMR is defined as the amount of calories your body will burn in a 24 hour period laying at rest but awake. It's basically how many calories you burn in a day without doing anything but breathing.

The second step is to take your BMR and apply what is known as an activity factor. The activity factors are as follows:

Little or no exercise per week	=1.2
Light exercise, lightly active	=1.375
Moderate exercise, 3-5 times per week	=1.55
Highly active, intense workouts	=1.725
Laborious job, intense workouts, marathons	=1.9

Simply multiply your BMR by the activity factor that best describes your weekly routine and you will then have what is called your Total Daily Energy Expenditure (TDEE), or basically how many calories per day you body burns given a certain level of activity. Your TDEE is the amount of calories your body needs to maintain your current body weight, body fat and general health.

Let's take a look at an example. Mary is a 45 year old woman. She currently weighs 160 pounds, and has a sedentary desk job with little activity in her daily routine. She visits with a personal trainer and has her body fat percentage measured, and it comes up to be 26%. That means that 26% of her 160 pounds of body weight is body fat; the remainder of her weight is made up of muscle mass and critical body organs and tissue, like skin, bones, organs and blood vessels.

So, the first thing to do with this basic information is to convert her body weight to kilograms (Kg), since the Katch-McArdle formula is based on the metric system. We do that by dividing her body weight by 2.2:

160lb/2.2 = 72.7Kg.

We then apply her body fat ratio of 26% to divide her weight into two categories, (1) body fat in Kg and (2) lean body mass in Kg:

72.7 X .26 = 18.9 Kg of body fat

72.7 X .74 = 53.8 Kg of lean body mass
(the .74 is 74%, or 1-.26)

Then we plug in Mary's numbers to the Katch-McArdle formula:

370 + (21.6 X 53.8) = 1,532 (BMR)

So, Mary's BMR, or the amount of calories that her body burns in a 24 hour period without any activity at all is 1,532. Since Mary is sedentary, we will use an activity factor of 1.2:

1,532 X 1.2 = 1,838.4 (TDEE)

Finally, this tells us that Mary will burn approximately 1,838 calories per day with her current lifestyle. That also means that in order to maintain her weight, she needs to eat 1,838 calories. If she eats more, she will gain weight and body fat. If she eats less, she will lose weight and body fat.

Now, I am not telling you to count calories. We all know that counting calories is laborious, tedious and not a long-term strategy. I also am not telling you to simply restrict your calories to below your TDEE to lose weight, if it were that simple then all diets would work and all you would have to do is starve yourself to succeed. But you now know about the starvation response, and that the human body has a built-in defense mechanism to guard against severe restriction.

What I am telling you is that in order to gauge your caloric intake, you must become familiar with portions and calories as best you can. Read labels, measure food for a couple of days, write your daily food intake down in a journal for a week or two so that you can review what you've done. Be disciplined for long enough to learn approximately how many calories are in your favorite foods. After a short time, you will know how many calories are in an 8 oz. glass of skim milk or 2 pieces of whole wheat bread.

Also, rather than taking the approach of just eating less to be in a deficit beneath your TDEE, I am telling you to eat enough calories to meet or exceed your TDEE and BURN off the excess by increasing your activity level. Burning off stored body fat is a much more efficient and permanent way to lose body fat than trying to starve it off! You must aim for a higher activity factor number, like 1.55 or moderate exercise. When this number increases, your fat loss kicks in!

The last factor to consider with regards to customization is your current lifestyle. Remember this golden rule: do what works for you and don't go overboard trying to do everything perfectly. We do not live in a perfect world, and losing body fat and keeping it off is a lifestyle, not something temporary. If you are short on time, find the foods that work for you and the exercise plan that fits your schedule. If you can't stand to cook, find some local restaurants that serve healthy dishes. The bottom line is this: whatever you do, it must work for you; otherwise, you will stop.

LAW #5 – THE LAW OF ADJUSTING GRADUALLY

This is the final concrete law of losing body fat. Laws 1-4 are all critical to the process, but this final law will discuss the importance of taking action gradually. There are two ways in which you must use this law in your favor when progressing towards your goal. The first is related to your daily calories and the second is related to your exercise plan, which we will discuss later on.

<u>The Law of Adjusting Gradually</u> – *if you make big changes all at once and adjust your calories either up or down too fast, your body will react*

much too drastically. If you jump in to exercise too quickly and push too hard, your body will reject what you are doing. You must incrementally and systematically make change; it cannot be overnight.

First, let's look at making proper incremental adjustments to your daily caloric intake levels. If you are like most working people, you might skip breakfast, maybe take a light working lunch, and then gorge at dinner with one (maybe two) glasses of wine and then some late night snacking before crashing in bed. Sound familiar?

Or maybe you find yourself stopping at the drive thru at a fast food joint for a breakfast sandwich and coffee, snacking or "grazing" throughout the day on whatever you can find, wolfing down your lunch in between tasks and then more snacking, with a large dinner to end the day.

Fact: most Americans work very hard either at their job and/or raising their family and have little time or desire to stop and eat a well-balanced meal. What happens is either one of two things: (1) they forget to eat during the day and as a result fit all of their calories into one large meal, or (2) use constant eating and snacking as a way to get through their stressful days, without any regard to what they are putting in their bodies. A typical person might find that they are way below or way above their Total Daily Energy Expenditure (TDEE) on a daily basis. Either way, an adjustment must be made.

ADJUSTING FOR THE PROPER AMOUNT OF CALORIES

First, you must get an approximate idea of how many calories you take in each day, then bounce that number off of your TDEE calculation to see if you are consistently in a deficit or a surplus. **Note: both a surplus and a deficit can cause someone to gain and retain excess body fat. This is because a surplus obviously means that a person is ingesting more calories than they need per day, and a deficit means that the starvation response has kicked in and that person's metabolism is slower than a snail. Neither situation is a great place to be and can cause massive weight gain.

Next, depending on how large the difference is between your actual intake and your TDEE, you must correct that difference. Say for instance that Mary (from our previous example) has a TDEE of 1,838 calories per day, and she usually takes in about 1,300 calories per day, because she really only eats twice per day, lunch and dinner. That's about a 500 calories deficit per day. Mary is under eating! She is also having way too many calories in just two sittings, so almost all of her calories are getting stored as body fat. She has been in this pattern for so long that her metabolism is virtually dead and gone, and her 45 year old body is functioning more like that of a 65 year old.

If Mary followed the laws above without adjusting gradually, she would jump from 1,300 calories per day to 1,800 calories overnight, and guess what would happen to Mary? Because her metabolic rate is so low from "starving" herself though the years, those extra 500 calories per day would immediately shock her body into fat storage mode. Mary would gain weight, and very quickly determine that this plan does not work at all.

Instead, Mary is going to have to incrementally adjust to get to her daily goal. First, Mary could take the amount of calories she normally takes in now and split that approximate amount into three or four smaller meals. So, the total doesn't change just yet, but the principle of stoking the metabolism again by having smaller meals is her first step. After a couple of weeks of making that first adjustment, Mary could then increase the size of her small meals and snacks by just a few calories to start bringing her up to speed.

Now, I want to reinforce a point here. Mary, or anyone for that matter, does not need to get ultra-detailed in this process; it's not that exact. If it becomes a burden for you, you will stop and give up. Just use common sense. Eventually, by making small increases, Mary will find the level that works best and feels best for her. Use your gut instincts and listen to your body.

The same principle applies if Mary is overeating on a daily basis. If she cuts her calories drastically overnight, she will see an initial weight loss, but that is nothing more than some water weight and muscle loss. Very quickly, her body will catch up to a severe cut in calories, and her metabolism will slow dramatically in order to compensate. A much more effective method would be to cut calories by a small percentage per day and incorporate some basic principles, such as eating smaller meals more frequently. A conservative approach would be to cut the difference between your TDEE and your actual caloric intake by 20% every two weeks for ten weeks total.

No matter what scenario you find yourself in now, in order to make these changes and approach them correctly, you must have patience and take the time to adjust slowly and gradually, otherwise disaster is right around the corner. Do not self-sabotage.

ADJUSTING FOR THE PROPER AMOUNT OF EXERCISE

If you are reading this book, chances are you have a love/hate relationship with exercise. You love how you feel when it's over, but you hate everything else about it. Some of you might even have a hate/hate relationship with exercise. The bottom line is this: your success depends on both your nutrition changes as well as a sound exercise plan. I'll explain a little later how you can make exercise simple and fun (and effective!), but for now just know that it must be a part of your plan.

If you are sedentary now, do not worry! Most of the clients I have worked with came to me having been inactive for quite some time. The good news is, in order to burn more calories per day than you do now, you don't need to go crazy with an overwhelming exercise program. Anything you do that is active is more than nothing. The other good news is that you can stick to things you enjoy, like walking, hiking, playing with your children or taking a family bike ride. You must start small. Have you ever known someone close to you that starts up an exercise program right after New Year's Day and hits the gym hard, only to not be able to walk for a week? Such methods are not very effective.

Start small, increase gradually as you become more fit and

comfortable with moving again, and remember to stick to activities that you enjoy! Otherwise, you will lose motivation quickly and eventually quit.

MANAGING YOUR EXPECTATIONS

One of the hardest parts of dieting and exercising to lose body fat is that we want the results YESTERDAY! We live in an on-demand world! The results can't come fast enough. Have you ever witnessed the gym rush that happens each year after January 1st? It's like the gym is giving away free money; everyone seems to make the same resolution and get started right away with best intentions. But what happens come February 1st? A mere 31 days later, 90% of those same people have quit. The gym is now a ghost town with just the regulars again. Why? Because the "Resolutioners" didn't see the overnight transformation they were hoping for, so they were convinced that nothing was working.

If you've ever been guilty of this, it's okay. I don't blame you at all. Why wouldn't you think that it would be an overnight transformation? The answer is that ads can be very convincing and misleading. The label on diet pills will promise you fast results. The nice guy on the infomercial will say the same thing, but you know deep down inside that those messages are lies. Most of the clients I have worked with admitted to me that they knew in their heart of hearts that nothing replaces good old hard work and discipline.

So, what can you expect if you are doing things correctly and following a lifestyle plan that is destined to be permanent? Are you ready for the brutal truth? The answer is: NOTHING! At least not at first. Let me explain. I've worked with hundreds of clients who saw literally no change in their appearance or their weight for the first month of working out and watching their nutrition! No change! In a whole month! Does that happen all of the time? No. But it does happen quite often.

Other times I have worked with clients that have seen drastic changes in just a couple of weeks. Does that happen all of the time? No. The point is that every person is different, with different metabolisms and health histories and physical abilities. The beginning results of a new lifestyle are totally unpredictable. Sometimes it takes a considerable amount of time to correct a lifetime of bad habits and yo-yo dieting. There are so many variables that can determine the speed of your success. I often remind my clients that they did not get to be 50 pounds too heavy overnight, so why would they expect to lose it overnight?

What happens all too often is this: someone will decide to make some changes, whether it's eating better or working out or both, and within 1-2 weeks they give up because it hasn't produced a result yet. In reality, a lot is happening to that person's internal bodily functions, but all that person cares about is the number on the scale. So they quit. Sound familiar? It probably does because most Americans are scaled-obsessed. Again, this is not your fault; we've been brain washed to think this way by the same companies that advertise for weight loss solutions. Why do we care about the number on the scale so much? Because we can see it and measure it and it's easily accessible information.

But does that number really matter? Would you care if you weighed 170 pounds but were a size 4? Men, would you really care if your scale told you that you were 220 pounds but you fit into size 32 pants? Most of my clients answered "No" to that question when asked. All that should matter is how you look and feel; that's the bottom line. The scale will never tell you how much muscle mass you have, or how much water weight you are retaining. That is why a scale is severely flawed. It is only measuring total weight, not the breakdown of that total weight into fat pounds and muscle pounds.

As for expectations over time, the truth is this: you cannot expect more than two pounds of body fat lost per week. Most times, my clients lost an average of one pound of body fat per week. I know that doesn't sound like much, but over the course of one year that equals 52 pounds! And imagine losing that fat permanently! Let's look at some simple math to illustrate this point:

There are 3,500 calories in one pound of body fat. Yes, 3,500.

I told you about the Law of the Calorie Deficit/Surplus earlier in this chapter, so you understand that you must burn 3,500 calories in a deficit in order to lose one whole pound of fat. That's a lot! So, let's say on a given day you stay consistent with your eating and you get in a good workout, and you end up 500 calories below your Total Daily Energy Expenditure (TDEE). Good for you; that is not easy! It gets even harder because you need to do that for seven straight days without one slip-up in order to lose one pound...ugh! If you're really working hard and burning a lot of calories each day, you might even be 1,000 calories below your TDEE, which if done for an entire week will yield just a two pound loss. That seems like a lot of hard work for not much of a payoff.

I am going to stop here and answer the question you might be thinking: "But John, when I dieted in the past, I lost 10 pounds in the first week! How can that be?" Here's the difference: I am not talking about losing *weight*, I am talking about losing BODY FAT! There is a big distinction between the two. When you have dieted in the past, you may very well have lost 10 pounds on the scale in that first week, but I'm willing to bet that 10 pounds was not all body fat, maybe not even any of it! The fact is, when you cut calories very drastically, especially carbs, your body loses mostly water weight at first, and it shows on the scale. To actually lose body fat, you need to burn 3,500 calories below your TDEE <u>without</u> sacrificing your metabolism. Otherwise, your weight loss will be nothing more than a loss in water weight and muscle tissue. That is what the next chapter is all about – your metabolism and how to ignite it.

RAPID RECAP

The 5 Concrete Laws of Losing Body Fat

1. <u>The Law of the Calorie Deficit/Surplus</u> – If you eat more than your body needs, you will gain weight. If you eat less than your body needs, you will lose weight.

2. <u>The Law of Portions</u> – You can eat what you want as long as it's small enough. On the flipside, if you eat too

much of anything, it will get stored away as body fat, even the good stuff! Portion control and spreading out your calories is a must!

3. The Law of Activity (You Need to MOVE!!!) – Burn off excess body fat. Do not try to starve it off. In order to burn more than you eat, you need activity and exercise. Otherwise, starving off the calories invokes the starvation response, which slows down the metabolism.

4. The Law of Customization – We are all unique. We all have different caloric needs, as well as limits to our level of change we can make. Use calculation and your common sense to find what works for you. Any cookie-cutter plan may have some good points, but everyone needs to be specific to their own situation.

5. The Law of Adjusting Gradually – Wherever you are now, do not make drastic changes overnight; you will shock your body. Change incrementally to get to an ideal level of calories and exercise. You must accept realistic expectations, and do not fall victim to a diet that promises huge losses in weight. Look at your change as a lifestyle (marathon) rather than a quick fix (sprint).

CHAPTER 5:

The 10 Undisputable Keys to Stoking Your Metabolic Fire Inside

"We never repent of having eaten too little."
- Thomas Jefferson

When it all boils down, the one and only true thing that you need to focus on while trying to burn body fat and transform your body is your metabolism. As you age, particularly once you hit 30, your metabolic rate naturally slows down year after year. That is a fact. Also, if you have ever been on the diet rollercoaster ride of gaining and losing weight over and over again through the years, than you know full well that each time you repeat that cycle, it gets a little tougher to lose the weight, and when you gain it back it seems to just reappear overnight.

This slowdown of your metabolism is very common. Each time you go on a diet, you almost always invoke the starvation response because you have chosen to cut your calories way below your daily maintenance level, or Total Daily Energy Expenditure (TDEE). As a result of the starvation trigger, your body slows down the rate at which it burns calories, causing most of what you eat to be stored as body fat.

When you eventually quit the diet, you begin eating normal or even excess quantities of food again, and most of what you eat gets stored away since your metabolism is in the basement! Thus, what you experience is the "rebound effect" or "yo-yo" or "rollercoaster" that we are all familiar with.

Repeating this process over and over is very debilitating on both your body and your mind, and is very frustrating. With traditional diets, the metabolism is the first thing to be sacrificed, when in fact it should be the one non-negotiable when living a healthy lifestyle. In this chapter, I will share with you the 10 undisputable keys to stoking your metabolic fire inside. Each of us has the capability of reviving and supercharging our metabolism, we just need to know how. Well, now you will know!

THE 10 UNDISPUTABLE KEYS TO STOKING YOUR METABOLIC FIRE INSIDE

Below are 10 tips on how to NEVER sacrifice your metabolism and also to reignite that internal furnace and keep it burning for life! Some of these keys you may have known or heard of before, and there may be many more effective ways other than these 10, but I can tell you that each one of these tips works extremely well…and none of these are what I would call "fads" or "gimmicks. These are just tried and true principles to live by:

1. *EAT!!!* – So your internal metabolic systems work much like a furnace. Food represents your fuel, or in this analogy, coal. If you don't eat food, your furnace stays cold and doesn't work. Food is not only fuel for your body; it's also food for your brain. If you eat whole foods spread out throughout the day, your furnace will always be burning hot and will metabolize any and all excess calories.

Too many traditional diets preach calorie cutting and restriction, as do many doctors that are trying to help their patients lose weight. I am telling you to EAT MORE! Can you believe it? Believe it! Now, don't take my advice out of context, there are limits, as we discussed earlier. Eat at, or slightly above, your TDEE, and burn off the excess with exercise and activity. This is rule #1 of never forfeiting your metabolism, and it is crucial.

2. *Eat 5-6 smaller meals/snacks through the day* – Most people have heard of this before, and this is one the techniques that stands the test of time. It is rule #2 for a reason; it is important! Imagine that furnace analogy for a minute, and visualize a pile of coal that represents your entire day's worth of food. If you typically only eat 1-2 large meals per day than that is much like shoveling that entire mound of coal into the furnace in one fell swoop. That furnace would certainly get very hot, but it would only last so long until it burned out and cooled off. The same goes for your metabolism.

A much more effective way at keeping your metabolic fire burning hot all day long is to shovel in that coal (food) gradually, and in smaller, spread-out increments. The human body typically digests a normal sized, well-balanced meal in about 2-3 hours time. So, have your 3 regular meals (breakfast, lunch and dinner) with 2-3 snacks in between spread out in 2-3 hour increments.

This accomplishes 2 things: (1) it keeps your metabolism high and churning/burning your calories, and (2) it naturally teaches you portion control because you will never be overly full or overly hungry to the point where you would binge.

3. *NEVER, EVER skip breakfast* – You must have heard this one for years growing up, "Eat a good breakfast!" Well, your mother was right all those years. A good breakfast does many things for you, but most importantly it gets your internal systems functioning properly and it jumpstarts your metabolism. Many of my clients have told me that they never eat breakfast either because they are not hungry in the morning or they are too busy. I tell them they are not hungry *because* they routinely skip breakfast, and as for being too busy – anyone can make time for a 5 minute breakfast if they really want to.

Think of your metabolism in the morning like a light switch. When you wake up, your body wants to turn on. Your body has been in a state of sleep where your metabolism has been virtually shut off. The only way to turn that light switch on is to eat. The longer you wait to do that, the longer your metabolism stays in the dark. So, ideally you should eat a well-balanced breakfast as soon as you can after waking.

You will also be more mentally alert and ready for your day. Think of all the times you skipped breakfast you were actually contributing to a slower state of mind through your day. Eating breakfast actually makes you more alert and clears your mind.

4. *Always get your protein* – When all else fails, you must be sure to include lean protein in your daily food intake. Lean proteins are the building blocks for healthy, strong and lean muscle mass, which is the most metabolically active tissue in your body. Muscle burns a lot of calories when it is up to par, and the stronger you are the more you'll burn through the day. Muscle tissue is made up mostly of proteins and water. When your muscles don't get the adequate amount of protein to stay strong and keep burning calories, you become a "catabolic." That's when your muscle eats away at itself to get the protein it's looking for...not good! That further contributes to a metabolic slowdown.

Also, lean protein that is found in foods such as eggs, fish, meats, chicken & poultry, beans, milk, and soy have what's called a "thermic effect" on the way your body digests food. What this means is that it takes a certain amount of energy for your body to digest food, and that energy equates to calories burned. It takes more energy, and thus more calories burned, to digest protein than any of the other two macronutrients, carbs and fats. So, you are actually burning more calories and speeding up your metabolism just by eating protein.

As for how much protein to get each day, that depends on who you talk to. My rule of thumb is to avoid over- or under-eating protein, and shoot to take in some protein with every meal and snack, rather than binging all at once. Generally, 20 grams per eating for a grown female is adequate, while 30-35 grams per eating for a grown male is a good ballpark number. Don't worry if this doesn't quite make sense; we'll talk about nutrient balancing in the next chapter.

5. *Carbohydrates are your friend, not your enemy* – Over the past 15 years or so, carbohydrates have received more bad press than imaginable. Suddenly, carbs are the enemy, and low-carb or even no-carb diets have become extremely popular. The Atkins and South Beach diets have convinced many people that carbs are the reason people gain and keep excess body fat.

I am here to tell you that carbs are one of your best friends! They are not only vital to your daily health, but they can also help you to lose body fat. There certainly are some bad carbs out there as well, and most times the problem lies in two areas: (1) proper portion of the carbs, and (2) differentiating the good carbs from the bad carbs.

There are many classifications of carbs, from low glycemic to high glycemic, simple and complex, refined, starchy and fibrous. We will talk more about carbs in the next chapter, so I will not go into detail about these classifications just yet. Just know this: carbs are your brain fuel as well as your energy source for your body. Without them, you cannot succeed at looking and feeling your best.

6. *Taper your calories and your carbs throughout the day* – Since carbs are used primarily for fuel, it makes sense to eat more carbs early in the day when your body will actually burn them, and less at night when your body is winding down and getting ready for rest. Too often clients of mine would tell me that they would eat a late night snack or a very heavy dinner shortly before crashing for the night. The result: most of those calories, especially the calories from carb sources, get stored away as body fat because your mind and body shut down when you rest at night.

As a general rule, do not eat anything at least 3 hours before you are going to sleep. This will allow for the calories that your body hasn't used up yet to be used and for you to go to bed on an empty stomach. This eliminates any chance of excess calories being stored.

Also, your last meal or snack of the day should be smaller in size and calories than the rest of your meals throughout the day, and it should be minimal in carbs as well. This technique is called tapering, and it implies that your biggest meal of the day is breakfast, and subsequent meals and snacks get smaller throughout the day.

7. *Choose whole and natural foods* – This tip is simple. When eating or drinking anything, ask yourself the following question: "Did this come from the earth or a living thing on Earth and is it in its natural state? Or is this a man made food/drink?" If your answer is: "Yes, this is food that has not been tampered with and is how nature intended it to be," then you pass! Fortunately, this is not pass/fail, so not everything you eat or drink has to be perfectly from nature or a living animal.

Tom Venuto in his e-book, Burn the Fat, Feed the Muscle, has a section entitled the "A Food, B Food Lecture." In it, he explains the varying grades of foods based on how much or how little they are processed. For example, take an apple. An apple by itself is an A grade. It came from the Earth, hasn't been changed or processed and is filled with lots of nutrients and vitamins. Take that apple and make unsweetened apple sauce and you now have a B grade. Go ahead and turn that apple sauce into apple juice by adding water, it turns to a C. Sweeten the apple juice or apple sauce with man-made sugar, it becomes a D. And finally, turn that apple into an apple pie, full of fat and sugar and you've got yourself an F.

The same goes for any food or drink you enjoy. It is not simply an A or an F. There are many varying grades, and you want the majority of your choices to be A's, B's and some C's. The D's and F's must be consumed in moderation. An easy way to set yourself up to do this on a consistent basis is to grocery shop primarily on the outer edges of the store; that is where most of the perishable foods are sold. Perishables are good because they contain little or no preservatives. They're also higher in nutrients and will be better absorbed by your body. This leads to an increase in your metabolism and general health function.

Another quick test is to see what packaging your food comes in. If it is in a can or a box, typically it will have a longer shelf life, which means it was made in a factory. There are many B and C grade foods out there that come in such packaging, but not many A's. Choose these foods sparingly and always read the labels. If you see ingredients that you can't even pronounce, don't buy it.

Here are some additives and preservatives to avoid at all costs:

1. High Fructose Corn Syrup
2. Partially Hydrogenated Oils
3. Trans Fats
4. Sodium Nitrate & Nitrite
5. Food Colorings
6. Monosodium Glutamate (MSG)
7. Anything you can't pronounce

There are many others out there, but to reinforce simplicity, use your best judgment and seek out foods that are as close to their natural state as possible, and enjoy the foods that are not in moderation.

8. *Plan ahead* – A wise man once said to me, "You must live your life by the Rule of the 5 P's…Proper Preparation Prevents Poor Performance!" Many times people fail to eat properly throughout the day because they are too busy and unprepared. I understand this, truly I do. Raising a family, working a ton of hours, go go go! That is the society we live in, and it seems that the more productive we've become with technology improvements, the less time we have! My clients would always ask me, "How can you expect me to even have the 5 minutes needed to eat every 3 hours?" Or, "I hate to cook, so other than eating fast food what options do I have?"

The answer is to keep it simple and take a few minutes at the beginning of the day or the week and prepare for your hectic schedule. Here are some tips to making sure you are prepared for your new lifestyle eating pattern:

1. Preparing meals weekly is helpful. Cook a large portion of food on Sunday and pack leftovers into Tupperware for the rest of the week.

2. If you cook daily or someone in your household does, cook a large dinner with plenty leftover, and pack the rest for tomorrow's lunch.

3. Set a reminder in your Outlook calendar to eat every 3 hours. Having a quick reminder pop up in front of you during work will help you to not miss meals/snacks.

4. Use meal replacement supplements to fill the mid-morning and afternoon gaps instead of heading to the vending machine. We'll talk about supplements a little later, but for now just know that the right supplements can be very convenient and help you to succeed.

5. Have portable foods at the ready. If you are constantly on the go, seek out foods that you can take with you in the car or running errands. Fruits are a great choice for this tactic.

6. Never leave home without water! Too many people are walking around each day slightly dehydrated. Tap water is fine, just fill up a cool thermos and off you go.

7. Plan your day in your head. Know what you wish to accomplish today for your eating habits, visualize it, and then make it a reality. Many of my clients never even thought about their eating habits prior to changing their lifestyle, but when it becomes a daily priority, you are more vested in your own success.

Planning ahead is a great technique with anything you do in life, whether it's work, your family, hobbies, or even your health. You must devote some time to draw out and execute your plan. Otherwise you will be inconsistent day after day.

9. *Enjoy "FREE" meals and follow the 90 Principle* – Life is too short. We all need to enjoy the things that we love most, and if you're anything like me, food is one of my biggest loves. Without this key concept, this entire plan will ultimately blow up in your face. "Deprivation" and "restriction" are negative words from my perspective. "Moderation" is a much better word, and can be used to your advantage. In order to stay sane when watching what you eat and changing your lifestyle, there must be some rewards that come with no guilt.

Here's a way to go about this rule systematically. Each week, schedule some "free" meals that you would really like to have, and plan for them. I use the word "free" with my clients rather than "cheat" because cheating implies that you are doing something wrong and terrible. Free meals are just the opposite; they are good for you mentally and they keep you satisfied and on track. You should never feel guilt or shame from enjoying a free meal. If you mentally prepare for these free meals and even go so far as scheduling them, then you will have something to earn through the week and you can look forward to your treat. My clients generally would have their free meals on a Friday or Saturday night, or maybe even a Sunday brunch.

Another great principle to live by is the 90 Principle. What this states is that over the course of a given week, if you are truly eating five to six smaller meals/snacks per day that equals to about 40 times per week that you will be eating food. Being strict 100% of the time is not realistic nor is it healthy for your wellbeing, so I preach to my clients to live by the 90 Principle, or have 10% of your meals/snacks that are FREE! That's four to five free meals per week.

Now don't go too crazy on the free meals, it certainly can be abused very easily. Use your best judgment, but don't hold back on your food choices. Just watch the portions, if you are going to enjoy pizza, have two or three slices with zero guilt. Just don't have the whole pizza!

10. *Cycle your calories using the Zig-Zag Method (THIS IS POWERFUL!!!)* – The Zig-Zag Method, or calorie cycling, is a technique that has been used by bodybuilders and athletes for many decades, and it is simply the most powerful way to rev up your metabolism while shedding pound after pound of excess body fat. It is even effective for anyone that might be stuck at a plateau. It is very simple, yet so powerful when done right that I am amazed that not many people know about it. Bodybuilders use this technique because they are the leanest people on Earth.

The basics of it are this: creating a calorie deficit, whether through calorie restriction or through burning off excess calories with exercise (much more effective!), can take its toll after a prolonged period. It's simply not good to always be in a calorie deficit, because you now know that your metabolism slows down eventually if you are in it too long. The Zig-Zag method corrects this slight problem by revving up your metabolism every so often to keep your internal furnace burning. What you do is systematically up your food intake on certain days of the week to make sure that your metabolism spikes up and corrects itself from being in a deficit for a few days.

There are many ways to cycle your calories, but I will give you the most common and basic example so that you have somewhere to begin. The easiest place to begin is to start with your Total Daily Energy Expenditure (TDEE) level, which was calculated in the previous chapter. If you choose to cut your calories just a bit to create a deficit, use a 15%-20% cut and don't cut any more than that. Plan on that level of calories for about 3 days, then on the 4th day, spike your calories back up to your TDEE level or even just above it by 15%-20%. This is a 3:1 cycle, or 3 low and 1 high, and is a great place to get started on the Zig-Zag Method.

Other ratios that work for others are a 3:2 or even a 3:3 ratio. Experiment and customize based on what works for you. Again, if you write down everything you eat for a week or two and make it a behavior of reading labels and learning the basics about the foods you love, you'll get the hang of this without having to always measure and weigh your food and count calories.

You shouldn't use this technique all of the time, as your body will adapt and get used to any pattern. However, as a general rule, I coach my clients to use calorie cycling for twelve weeks at a time, then take a month off where you eat basically at your TDEE level for maintenance and to regulate your system.

RAPID RECAP

The 10 Undisputable Keys to Stoking Your Metabolic Fire Inside

1. EAT!!! Restricting your calories and starving yourself is over!
2. Eat five to six smaller meals/snacks through the day.
3. NEVER, EVER skip breakfast.
4. Always get your protein.
5. Carbohydrates are your friend, not your enemy.
6. Taper your calories and your carbs throughout the day.
7. Choose whole and natural foods.
8. Plan ahead.
9. Enjoy "FREE" meals and follow the 90 Principle.
10. Cycle your calories using the Zig-Zag Method.

CHAPTER 6:

The Nutrient Balancing Principle: The Truth About Protein, Carbohydrates and Fats

"Whatever will satisfy hunger is good food."
- Chinese Proverb

"The belly is ungrateful – it always forgets we already gave it something."
- Russian Proverb

Have you ever tried to count calories? How about breaking out a food scale and measuring your portions? Don't get me wrong, these behaviors are great and have tremendous value, but after a while it can get very tedious and start to feel like a second job.

Also, most people have no idea what a "balanced" meal really consists of, nor do they know if the portion is correct or what factors go into having a meal that is well balanced. With all of the bad information out there, it is easy to see how someone could be confused. For that reason, the Nutrient Balancing Principle exists:

The Nutrient Balancing Principle – *in order to optimize fat burning and general health, one must properly balance meals to include lean protein, complex and/or natural carbohydrates, and healthy unsaturated fats in a manner that supports a balanced ratio, such as 3:2:1 carbs:proteins:fats.*

The goal of this chapter is threefold: (1) to explain proteins, carbs and fats into simple terms so that you can learn why each of these nutrients is critical to your health and wellness, as well as achieving your fast loss goal, (2) to teach you how to properly balance your meals and to discuss the importance of combining certain nutrients in order to help you reach your goal, and (3) to finally learn how to give up counting calories the simple way so you can continue to live your life without the hassle.

MACRONUTRIENTS: THE BIG THREE

In the world of food and drink, there are two categories of nutrients that virtually all foods fall into when broken down: (1) micronutrients, which are all of the vitamins, minerals and enzymes of a food on a very specific level, such as Vitamin C, and (2) macronutrients, or the Big Three, which are divided into three categories: proteins, carbohydrates and fats. Here I will break out each of these three macronutrients so that you will know why each of them is vital to your success, as well as how to combine them to really get the results you need! I will not cover micronutrients, for I am sure that you don't care to know the inner workings of the B Vitamins or why Folic Acid works the way it does. For that type of in-depth analysis, please refer to a scientific journal on nutrition. For now, just make sure you get a good multi-vitamin/mineral supplement, and we'll talk about that in a later chapter on supplements.

In this program, you will be using the 3:2:1 ratio of balancing your meals, and that translates to 3 (50% carb): 2 (35% protein): 1 (15%fat), which is a basic yet very healthy and powerful way to balance your nutrients. Keep this in mind while reading this chapter and when you calculate your breakdown:

1 gram of protein equates to 4 calories

1 gram of carbohydrate equates to 4 calories

1 gram of fat equates to 9 calories

Remember, calories are just a way of measuring your nutrients and how much energy is needed to process those nutrients and stay alive through the day. See how fat grams are more than double the calories of proteins and carbs? That's why so many foods that are high in fat are also high in calories.

PROTEIN – THE KING OF ALL NUTRIENTS

As I stated in Chapter 5, if all else fails, always get your protein! Protein is critical to your health and to losing body fat simply because it is the building block for your entire body. All of the muscle tissue in your body, your bones and organs, and even the hair on your head is made up of protein components. Your body is made up of anywhere from 70%-80% water, and protein is the next most abundant tissue in your body. It is essential! The most important role of protein is to provide your body with muscle mass, so that you can function properly on a daily basis, including walking, running, sitting, standing, breathing and any kind of movement you can think of. Sound important? It is!

Proteins are essentially made up of amino acids, which are the building blocks of protein. Amino acids can be divided into two categories: (1) essential amino acids or (2) non-essential amino acids. The first group, the essential amino acids, consists of those aminos that cannot be produced by your body naturally and must be provided through food. The list of essential aminos is as follows:

Histidine
Isoleucine
Leucine
Lysine
Methionine
Phenylalanine
Threonine
Tryptophan
Valine

The second group, or non-essential aminos, consists of those aminos that your body naturally produces and does not need from food, and that list is as follows:

Alanine

Arginine

Asparagine

Aspartic Acid

Cysteine

Glutamic acid

Glutamine

Glycine

Proline

Serine

Tyrosine

Any protein that contains all of the essential and non-essential amino acids is called a "complete" protein, meaning that it is not missing any of these amino acids. Examples of complete proteins include meat, fish, poultry, eggs, milk, cheese and whey. A great way to remember what a complete protein might be is to ask yourself if the protein source comes from a living animal or fish or is a byproduct of such. For example, milk is not a living animal, but it does come from a living animal, a cow. A peanut, however, is not from an animal or fish source, but it does contain protein; therefore, it would be classified as "incomplete."

In regard to losing body fat, protein is important because it strengthens your muscles, which in turn burn more calories throughout the day. Also, as stated before, protein has a "thermic" effect on digestion. When you eat protein, especially complete proteins, your body requires more heat and energy to digest that protein, which speeds up your metabolic rate and burns more calories! Also, complete proteins are responsible for building muscle, which in turn increases your metabolism (again, burns more calories too!).

Your goal is to have a complete protein with as many meals and snacks as you can. Because not all proteins are complete, you can combine certain foods that have many of the amino acids listed above to fill in the other food's gaps. For instance, peanut butter is missing some of the essential amino acids so it is not a complete protein. Whole grains found in bread are similar in that the protein content is incomplete; however, if you spread peanut butter on whole grain bread, that combination creates a complete protein by joining all of the amino acids in both foods. The bread "completes" the peanut butter! Other examples of incomplete proteins being combined to create a complete protein include tofu and rice, yams and green peas, and hummus on whole grain crackers. This is an important strategy, especially for vegetarians that do not ever get complete proteins from animal sources.

HOW MUCH PROTEIN DO I NEED?

So how much protein do you need? That is a controversial question. The National Research Council, which sets the Recommended Daily Allowances (RDA's) for nutrient and food consumption, will tell you one thing, fitness professionals will tell you another, and Joey Muscles at your local gym might offer yet another perspective. There is no conclusive research that offers a definitive answer for this ongoing question, but a very effective way to determine the right amount of protein is to apply a percentage of protein to your total calories per day.

In this program, the ideal percentage of your daily calories to apply to your protein intake is approximately 35%. This will apply to most people, but of course you must find what works best for you. I can tell you from my own experience that having somewhere around 35% of my total calories come from protein sources has yielded amazing results, not only for me, but for hundreds of my clients.

In order to do that, you must refer to your Total Daily Energy Expenditure (TDEE) calculation from before as your starting point. Remember, your TDEE is the amount of calories that you will burn in a 24 hour period including all of your activity. From that number, we will now figure out your 3:2:1 ratio of carbs:proteins:fats.

Example

TDEE = 1,700 (typical adult female profile)

3:2:1 ratio, or 50%:35%:15% (carbs:proteins:fats)

Step 1 1,700 X .50 = 850 calories from carbs per day, divided by 4 calories per gram of carb = 213 grams of carbs per day

1,700 X .35 = 595 calories from protein per day, divided by 4 calories per gram of protein= 149 grams of protein per day

1,700 X .15 = 255 calories from fat per day, divided by 9 calories per gram of fat = 28 grams of fat per day

Step 2 Divide the number of carbs:proteins:fats grams per day into 5-6 meals:

213/6 = 35g of carbs per meal/snack

149/6 = 25g of protein per meal/snack

28/6 = 5 g of fat per meal/snack

Now you have the approximate amount of carbohydrates, protein and fat per day and per meal using the 3:2:1 ratio.

CARBOHYDRATES – HIGH OCTANE FUEL FOR THE BODY AND MIND

Think of your body like it is a car. Would your car run if you didn't have any gas in it? If you had a high performance sports car (or wanted one) would that run best on low octane fuel? Would your sedan even start if you put diesel in it? NO! The same goes for your body. Think of food as your premium fuel to provide you energy throughout the day and during activity. Without food, or without the right kinds of food, your body will putt-putt through the day, or even break down. Also, carbs are brain food. Without carbs, your brain moves at a snail's pace. Have you ever skipped breakfast and felt a little slow? Physically and mentally? Nine times out of ten that is due to a carb deficiency.

There is a lot of confusion when it comes to carbs: "Are they good? Are they bad? Am I carb sensitive? All carbs are the same! I don't need carbs, so I'll just cut them out." Well, no more confusion; I will lay it all out for you so that you know just how important carbs are for your fat loss success and for your health. What you will learn is that the good carbs will be your new best friend. Those carbs will help you to lose body fat and stay energized constantly without hitting the 3pm wall. But, I will also address the bad carbs, because they do exist. The bad ones will do just the opposite; they'll cause you to go in the wrong direction and not only lead to you to keeping stored body fat but gaining more as well.

THE TYPES OF CARBOHYDRATES

There are two basic types of carbohydrates: simple and complex. These two types of carbs can then be categorized as (1) fibrous or starchy, (2) high or low glycemic and (3) natural or refined. To start, we will discuss the two major types, and then I will breakdown the glycemic index and the difference between fibrous, starchy, refined and natural carbs.

1. *Simple carbohydrates* – these are your fruits (or fructose), table sugar (sucrose), or sugar found in milk (or lactose). Simple carbs are basically one or two simple sugar molecules. The main concern with simple carbs has to do with your blood sugar. Because these carbs are simple, they are digested rapidly and cause a sudden spike in your blood sugar. As a result, your body releases insulin, which is a hormone that washes away the blood sugar, leaving you feeling like you've "crashed" since your blood sugar (or glucose) is now gone.

Why is this not good? Well, insulin promotes fat storage in your body. It also prevents fat burning. This is partly why carbs have gotten such a bad rep. If you take in a large amount of simple carbs throughout the day, your blood sugar levels are on a roller coaster ride and continue the downward spiral of increased fat storage. Does this mean that fruit is bad for you? Not at all! Any simple carb that can be further defined as "natural," meaning that it comes to your plate in its natural state, is very good for you. For instance, take an apple. That is a simple carb. In its natural state, that apple offers many nutrients, antioxidants and enzymes, as well as some energy.

However, simple carbs that are natural must be properly portioned. Too many simple carbs, even from natural sources, can cause similar results to that of regular table sugar, which is a "refined" simple carb. Refined means that a food is a man made product and not provided by nature. So, when choosing simple carbs for your fat loss plan, keep them to a minimum (2-3 per day) and always seek out the natural sort rather than the refined sort.

2. *Complex carbohydrates* – these are your carbs that take longer to digest since complex carbs are made up of thousands of sugars linked together, such as potatoes, rice, vegetables, oats, grains and beans. The complex carbs can be natural or refined as well, and also can be divided into two further categories, fibrous or starchy.

Complex carbs that are natural are obviously the better choice over refined because you now know that refined foods are man-made and tampered with, and the nutrients and enzymes in those foods are killed off in the course of processing them in the factories. Again, the best question to ask yourself when you are consuming a carbohydrate food is, "Is this food in its most natural state as nature intended it to be, or was this food processed and packaged?" The least refined carbs you can find are the best for your fat loss success, since you will be getting the most nutritional benefit which leads to your body performing at its peak.

When a carbohydrate is refined, not only does it lose its nutritional value, it also takes on characteristics of a simple carb, which has much more of a drastic impact on your blood sugar levels and promotes fat gain and storage. Examples of refined carbs include enriched white flour, regular semolina pasta, enriched rice and breads, crackers that are not 100% whole wheat and regular pretzels. These refined carbs should be consumed at a minimum to maximize results.

So, assuming you choose mostly natural complex carbs during the day, those foods can either be starchy or fibrous. Starch is basically a plant's energy, and carbs that are considered starchy include wheat, potatoes, grains, rice, oats and beans, among others. This category is where you will be getting most of your body's energy and your brain's fuel throughout the day. These foods are very dense in nutrients and energy, and are completely digested by the body to be used.

The other type of complex carbohydrates is fibrous carbs. Basically, these are your fresh vegetables. Your fibrous carbs, or vegetables, are a critical factor in your success because they are typically very low calorie, very high in vitamins and minerals, and the fiber that is present in these foods helps to not only curb your hunger, but it also slows down the digestion of your other foods, keeping your blood sugar levels steady without the peaks and valleys that can cause fat storage. Fiber is a wonderful thing! Unfortunately, too many of us do not get nearly enough fiber because so much of our food choices are heavily processed and have virtually no fiber content. That is why you must include fresh vegetables in their natural state into your daily routine. Some examples of fibrous carbs include tomatoes, zucchini, mixed greens, broccoli and spinach, among many others.

THE GLYCEMIC INDEX

The glycemic index (GI) has gained much popularity as well as criticism over the past decade. The basic function of the GI is to quantify the speed at which a carbohydrate breaks down into glucose, or blood sugar. Why is this important? Well, remember that when your blood sugar spikes quickly from consuming a simple carb, an overage of the hormone insulin is released to wash away the blood sugar, and then without blood sugar you feel a "crash." That insulin hormone promotes fat storage, and repeating that cycle many times over and over creates a fat storing atmosphere that is hard to correct.

So, the glycemic index was created in order to classify carbs into low or high glycemic foods so that you know which ones to avoid and which ones to seek out. This index was originally used by diabetics, since someone with diabetes needs to monitor their blood sugar levels in order to keep their condition in check. And then the GI went mainstream, and "glycemic" has been a buzzword ever since.

The GI has many benefits, but is also severely flawed, so let's look at the truth behind the concept. The GI ranks every carbohydrate food on a scale from 0 to 100, with 0 being the value that represents low glycemic foods that have virtually no impact on your blood sugar levels, and 100 representing high glycemic foods that have a drastic impact on spiking your blood sugar levels very quickly. The index also assumes that you are ingesting these carb foods when you are completely fasted (empty stomach and digestive tract) and that you are eating only that carb food alone, no protein, fat or additional vegetables. According to the index, any carbohydrate with a GI value of 70 or above is considered to be high, 56 to 69 is medium, and 55 and under is low.

The reason these assumptions are misleading is that very rarely will you be totally fasted, since on this program you will be eating approximately every 3 hours, and you will never be eating just a carb food by itself since this program teaches you how to balance your meals properly using the 3:2:1 ratio of carbs:proteins:fats. For instance, when you use the 3:2:1 ratio for your meals, the protein, healthy fat and fiber that you include with your complex carbs all help to slow down the rate at which the carbs are converted into blood sugar, essentially turning a high glycemic food into a lower glycemic food.

Combining your nutrients is one of the most important techniques you can master in order to lose body fat and keep it off. For example, watermelon has a glycemic value of 72, which is considered to be high on the index. So, hardcore followers of the GI will tell you that watermelon is bad for you and to stay away from it forever. Or, regular shredded wheat cereal has a GI value of 83, or very high. Should you not eat shredded wheat in the morning for that reason? Well, if you ate the watermelon as a part of a well balanced meal that also included some peanut butter on 100% whole wheat toast, then the GI value decreases significantly because the healthy fat, protein and fiber slow down the absorption rate of the watermelon. Or, if you have the shredded wheat with skim milk, a banana and some walnuts all mixed together you get the same scenario. Potatoes and carrots are also high on the GI; are they bad for you? Do they make you fat? I think you now know how to use your own common sense and make good decisions based on good information. Balancing your meals makes much of the GI's claims inaccurate.

HOW MANY CARBS DO I NEED?

Refer to my example above in the section on protein consumption; you will find that on average, your proper carb intake each day should fall somewhere near the 50% mark of your total calories. That would follow the 3:2:1 ratio, which provides you with the right amount of energy for your entire day as well as the correct amount of protein to build and maintain your muscle mass.

The fact is that 50% is not a perfect number for everyone. You must find what works best for you. I can tell you that most of my clients saw amazing results in losing body fat permanently by adopting the 3:2:1 ratio. Does that mean some people are not "carb sensitive"? By all means, no. Does that also mean that certain people don't need any more than 50% of the calories to come from carbs? Absolutely not. There are many people that would be characterized as carb sensitive, and if you feel that you are one of those people, my recommendation would be to drop your carb intake to no less than 40%, and make up the difference with an increase in protein and healthy fat. As for people who need more carbs, like distance athletes or manual laborers, I would recommend an increase in carbs to about 60% to compensate for the amount of energy you need daily. Again I stress the importance of experimenting a bit and finding what works best for you.

FATS: NOT ALL FATS ARE CREATED EQUAL

Over time, fats have been both hated and loved. In the 80's, fats were the most evil of evils. Everything was low fat or no fat, and fats were thought of to be the sole reason for heart attacks, strokes, high cholesterol and being overweight. Then came the 90's, when carbs got their bad rep and very quickly many people were becoming wise to the many benefits of fats. Today, there is still much confusion when I ask my clients about fats and carbs. You are now the expert on carbs, so let's talk about fats to clear up any doubts you may have.

Here is the truth: there are "good" fats, and there are "bad" fats. Think of a wide spectrum, with two ends that represent the best of the best and the worst of the worst. That is what the world of fats is like. The "bad" fats really are terrible, and can cause your arteries to clog, can contribute to you having a stroke or heart attack, and maybe even kill you. That's pretty far down the extreme end of the spectrum. However, on the other side of that spectrum are the "good" fats. These fats can actually help you to burn fat, can increase your energy, keep you looking and feeling young and improve the way your organs function. There is no real middle ground here, which is why so many only focus on the negative impacts of the "bad" fats and forget or ignore the many wonderful benefits of the "good" fats.

Most of us have tried a low fat or fat free diet at some point. In fact, in this program I am recommending only 15% of your calories to come from fat sources. That 15% goes along way though, especially if it's from the "good" fats. On a very low fat or no fat diet, some major issues arise that cause you to gain and keep body fat. First, because fats are higher in calorie (9 calories per gram) than protein or carbs (4 calories per gram), any extremely low fat regimen is inherently going to be low in total calories, thus invoking the starvation response. Secondly, if you have no fat to help with digestion, your insulin sensitivity to carbs will be much higher, causing you to become "carb sensitive."

The bottom line is that fats are in our lives for a purpose. They not only protect our internal organs and help us to maintain healthy skin, hair and nails, but fats are even a big part of your success at losing body fat. So what is the difference between a "bad" fat and a "good" fat?

I will keep this as simple as I can. I will classify all saturated fats and trans fats as "bad" fats. Some foods that are natural, such as eggs or red meat, contain saturated fats, so I don't mean to say that eggs and meats are bad for you. But, you should keep the egg yolks and the red meat consumption to a moderate level and don't overdo it. Trans fats are those saturated fats that have been processed further and are in many manmade foods, such as margarine. Foods high in saturated fats and/or trans fats include the following:

Butter

Margarine

Doughnuts

Cookies

Hydrogenated oils

Pastries

Full-fat cheeses

Whole milk

Shortening

Cooking lard

Fried foods

These foods should be used in strict moderation, and should not be a regular part of your nutrition plan to lose body fat.

Unsaturated fats and essential fatty acids (EFA's) are the "good" fats. Most foods you buy have a breakdown on the label of the total fat amount into saturated and unsaturated fats. Seek out those foods that are a healthy source of unsaturated fats and EFA's. A breakdown of these foods is included in the last section of this chapter. These foods should be a regular part of your daily nutrition plan. Believe it or not, taking in healthy fats can help you lose fat. I know, it seems crazy, but it's true. So don't ignore fat or assume all fats are the same; clearly they are not.

THE DOUBLE WHAMMY

There is a double whammy out there that will prevent you from succeeding more than any other type of food: it is the combination of saturated fats with refined carbs. These types of food include pizza, pastries, Chinese take-out, full-fat lasagna and ice cream, among many others. Most of these foods have white flour, sugar, saturated fat and/or cream of some combination. These foods are to be used in strict moderation, and should be viewed as your "free" meals. Plan for these meals and enjoy them when you've earned them. Do not make them a daily occurrence. I know, it's the good stuff. But, if you are serious about your success, be aware of any food that has both refined simple carbs and saturated fats; it is a double whammy.

LEARN PORTIONS AND NEVER COUNT CALORIES AGAIN!

So far, we have discussed the importance of proteins, carbs and fats, and you are now the expert on the Big 3 macronutrients. You know how much of each macronutrient you will need per day. You also now know why it is critical to combine your nutrients to help you lose body fat and keep it off.

The last step in this chapter is to provide you with a simple way to stay within your calorie and nutrient targets without driving yourself crazy counting calories. Counting calories is very important to your success, at least for a small time, so that you can become familiar with just how many calories are in your favorite foods. What I coach my clients to do is pay strict attention to calories and portions for 1-2 weeks at first, using the Internet or a calorie book as a guide. Write down your day's worth of food and drink, and have the discipline to start paying attention to calorie counts. Learn which foods are proteins, carbs and healthy fats. Before you know it, you've learned the basics so that you can make good decisions going forward, since most people tend to eat similar things each day.

Below is a simple list of the best foods you can eat to maximize your fat loss, separated by proteins, complex and simple carbs, and healthy fats. Next to each food you will find an approximate portion size for both adult males and females that will be your guide for portioning your meals. This list and the portions are based on an average adult male with a daily calorie goal (TDEE) of 2,400 calories and an average adult female with a daily calorie goal (TDEE) of 1,800 calories. Again, these are estimates, and every individual is different, but this is a great place to start as a resource.

Lean Proteins	Portion-Female	Portion-Male
Chicken and other poultry	4 oz.	6 oz.
Eggs and egg whites	1-2	2-3
Lean meats	4 oz.	6 oz.
Fish & shellfish	6 oz.	8 oz.
Skim milk	8 oz.	12 oz.
Low fat cottage cheese	6 oz.	10 oz.

Complex Carbs		
Brown rice	½ cup cooked	1 cup cooked
Potatoes and yams	½ portion	1 whole
Oatmeal	½ cup dry	1 cup dry
Whole grain bread	1 slice	2 slices

Whole wheat pasta	1 cup cooked	2 cups cooked
Legumes	½ cup cooked	1 cup cooked
Fresh vegetables	1-2+ cups dry	2-3+ cups dry
<u>Simple Carbs</u>		
Fresh fruits	1 piece	1 piece
Unsweetened fruit sauce	1 cup	2 cups
Fresh fruit juice	6 oz.	8-10 oz.
Unsweetened dried fruits	4 oz.	6 oz.
<u>Healthy Fats</u>		
Flaxseed and flaxseed oil	1 Tbsp.	2 Tbsp.
Olive oil	1 Tbsp.	2 Tbsp.
Nuts	1 oz.	2 oz.
Avocado	½ portion	1 whole
Fish and fish oils	1 Tbsp.	2 Tbsp.
Soybeans	½ cup	1 cup
Natural peanut butter	1 Tbsp.	2 Tbsp.

An ideal meal or snack would contain a lean protein from the list above, as well as a complex carb and a fruit or vegetable, with a healthy fat added in as needed. For example, a 6 oz. piece of salmon with ½ cup of brown rice and a salad with avocado is a perfectly well balanced meal. Remember to use spices to enhance flavor rather than butter or other types of fattening foods. Also, grilling, baking, sautéing and broiling are the best ways to prepare food, rather than frying. Keep to the general portions listed above, and once you learn what 6 oz. of fish or a cup of brown rice looks like, you'll never need to measure your food or count calories again! You'll be armed with the knowledge and discipline to make good decisions on your own.

RAPID RECAP

1. There are 3 major types of nutrients, called macronutrients. They are (1) protein, (2) carbohydrates and (3) fats.

2. Each macronutrient is critical to losing body fat, and combining the 3 to create a well balanced meal is best for results.

3. Protein is the most critical. It helps to build and retain muscle, increase your metabolism, and provide the thermic effect.

4. Carbs are your energy; without them your body is like a car without fuel.

5. Fats are essential, you must seek out healthy fats in avoid saturated fats and trans fats. By all means, avoid the double whammy!

6. Learn portions and calorie counts over the course of a couple of weeks so that you can use your knowledge to plan your meals and exercise portion control.

CHAPTER 7:

We Are ~~Human~~ Water Beings: The role of water (and its enemies) in your fat loss achievement

"In the world there is nothing more submissive and weak than water. Yet for attacking that which is hard and strong nothing can surpass it."
- Lao-Tzu

Our bodies are made up of about 70% water. I'm sure you've heard that before; it's no secret. Many people feel that we are a product of our Mother Earth, since our planet is also covered in approximately 70% water, and in order to survive the conditions here on Earth our bodies evolved over billions of years, bringing us to our current state of being.

Essentially, we are "water" beings, even more so than we are "human" beings. Water is what we are mostly made of, and we simply cannot survive very long at all without adequate amounts of water. People have proven throughout the years that a human being can survive on little or no food for as long as 2-3 weeks if faced with an extraordinary situation.

However, 2-3 days is the longest you could survive without water. Your muscles are made up mostly of water as is the blood running through your veins. Again, you probably already know this, so why am I dedicating an entire chapter to water?

Water is one of the most overlooked and underappreciated

factors when trying to lose body fat; however, obtaining the right amount of water each day could very well be the most powerful (and simple) way of losing your excess body fat and looking and feeling the way you want to! Also, it is vital to discuss some other liquid options that you may come in contact with each day and what the positive or negative effects can be on your progress from drinking such things as alcohol, coffee, soda, juice and sports drinks.

MOST OF US ARE DEHYDRATED

It is a sad fact that most of us walk around each day either slightly dehydrated or even dangerously dehydrated. Many people do not drink enough water, and as a result their bodies are not performing as they should. Partial or full dehydration causes headaches, fatigue, mental slowness, decreases in strength and endurance, and even an inability to lose body fat. Simply put, when your body is not getting enough water, it slowly shuts down.

The trouble is most people don't even recognize that they are dehydrated until it is too late. Some may never realize it. I have worked with so many clients that told me that the only water they get each day is whatever water is in their coffee. I honestly don't know how they have survived so long! The biggest mistake most people make is that they wait until they are thirsty to drink water, when in fact they are too late. If you wait for a sign, you missed the boat. Your body is already telling you that you are dehydrated.

WATER AND YOUR FAT LOSS GOAL

In regards to fat loss, water plays a significant role. In fact, it is so powerful that if you change only one thing in your lifestyle after reading this book, make that change be to drink the appropriate amount of water for you. This is because your water intake is the one factor that can trump all of the rest of the rules and principles you have learned thus far. If your body is dehydrated, nothing else matters in your quest to be lean and fit (and healthy!).

It works like this: First, your fat loss nutrition plan follows the 3:2:1 ratio of carbs:proteins:fats, which leads to about 35% of your calories coming from protein sources. You know that now. Because this program assumes that you are an active adult burning off stored fat calories rather than starving them off (we'll talk about exercise at the end), you need that protein to help build and maintain muscle mass. Having that amount of protein daily means that your kidneys will need that much more water intake to flush out toxins and waste matter. If you don't have adequate water intake, your body will naturally hold on to any water it has, much like the starvation response with food. When this happens, the kidneys can't work properly, and the toxins build up inside of you. As a result, your liver gets involved to help flush out the built up toxins. Your liver does many things, one of which includes burning stored body fat. When your liver is busy helping out your poor kidneys, it can't perform that function. You are in effect shutting down your body's ability to burn fat by being thirsty.

Second, because your muscles are the most metabolic tissue in your body and are made up of more than 70% water, they typically don't function properly when they are thirsty. Your muscles burn a lot of calories for you when they are hydrated, strong and well worked. Without the water they need to perform, they shut down. You literally are turning off the fat-burning ability of your muscles and contributing to further fat storage.

These are just a couple of examples of how your body does not operate at peak performance when you are short on water. Many of our internal functions rely on water in order to perform correctly and efficiently, including our digestion, our cardiovascular system, and our central nervous system. Without a positive water balance, you simply cannot reach your body's fat loss potential, nor can you be a healthy individual. In fact, when your body is short on water by just 10% of your body weight, it can be fatal. Also, your brain activity is slowed due to dehydration, causing you to make poor decisions and to operate sluggishly throughout the day. None of these symptoms lend themselves well to a healthy lifestyle, let alone burning fat.

HOW MUCH WATER DO I NEED?

Growing up we were all taught to have eight 8 oz. glasses of water per day, or 64 oz. per day. That is certainly a great place to start, and if most people stuck to that rule they'd be just fine. But that rule does not apply to everyone, especially active people. Again, we will go over your exercise plan in later chapters, but for now just assume that you are active. If you aren't now, you will be soon. You just wait!

Just like a solid nutrition plan, a person's water intake should be customized. There are more theories on water intake levels than you can imagine, and the most important thing to remember is to find what works best for you in your daily life. If you live in a hot climate, you will need more water than someone that doesn't. If you are a manual laborer, obviously your energy expenditure is greater than an office worker, and you will tend to sweat and release more water from your body. There are many factors, and you must consider all factors that relate to your daily routine.

To keep it simple, I use a guideline with my clients of starting with 64 oz. per day and keeping that range as a bare minimum, and then adjusting that figure based on just how many calories they expend in one day. As stated before, per ASCM guidelines, the least amount of calories an adult female should ever take in per day is 1,200 calories. So, if 1,200 calories is your Total Daily Energy Expenditure (TDEE), then start with 64 oz. of water per day. Remember, we calculated your TDEE in chapter 4. For every additional 400 calories your TDEE increases from 1,200, simply increase your daily water intake by 10 oz. This easy chart makes it easy for you to find your specific needs:

TDEE	Water (oz.) per day
1,200	64 oz.
1,600	74 oz.
2,000	84 oz.

2,400	94 oz.
2,800	104 oz.
3,200	114 oz.
3,600	124 oz.

Just like anything else, this is a general guide. Adjust up or down based on what works best for you. Contrary to popular belief, increasing your water intake will not make you feel bloated. It does just the opposite. You will find that your body is flushed out and functions very well when well hydrated. The only side effect here is that you might find yourself running to the bathroom more often than not, but if your water intake is far below these guidelines, you must commit to correcting this if you plan to succeed at losing body fat.

IS THERE SUCH THING AS TOO MUCH WATER?

So, can you overdo drinking water? In a word, yes! There is such a thing called water intoxication, and it can be fatal. This is very rare, but it can happen, especially when someone has over-exerted themselves and tries to replenish water by drinking excessive amounts very quickly. There have been some cases in the military or in sports where an individual will be faced with heat stress and/or overexertion which has lead to water intoxication cases. As for the normal everyday person, a good barometer to use is provided by the U.S. Army, which is 1-1 ½ quarts of water per hour and no more than 12 quarts per day, both at a maximum. Again, use your best judgment based on how much water your body can take without overdoing it.

IS TAP WATER OKAY OR SHOULD I DRINK BOTTLED WATER?

This question has been very controversial as of late, and it comes down to personal preference. In my own research, tap water in most cities and towns in America is fine for consumption. Maybe adding a simple filter to your tap to enhance the quality and eliminate any unwanted additives might be a safe option. Bottled water is great too since it is portable and if you happen to have a bottle of water with you, you're more likely to remember to drink water and stay hydrated.

There have been some studies showing that many of today's popular bottled water brands are actually more toxic then standard tap water. Some other studies will tell you that our tap water is highly contaminated, and to use a filter of some kind at all times. Again, it boils down to personal preference, and if need be do your own research and make that call.

Regardless of which source you get your water, just make sure you get it!

THE ENEMIES OF WATER

Water is your friend. It may even be your best friend. You need it to survive. Without it, you won't last long. Just like any great friend, water has its enemies. There are 5 key enemies of water: (1) soda, (2) alcohol, (3) sports drinks, (4) juices from concentrate, and (5) sodium. These bad guys will not only suppress your health, but totally inhibit your fat loss progress. Liquid calories always creep up on you, since they typically don't fill you up like food does, and most times liquid calories from drinks such as soda are extremely "empty" calories, offering little or no nutritional value. Let's talk about each of these villains and how they pertain to your fat loss program.

1. *Soda* – The problem with soda is that 99% of soda drinks that exist today are completely unnatural in every way. Regular sodas contain high amounts of manmade sugar, which have a large effect on your blood sugar levels, which contributes to fat storage. Also, the calories in soda add up in your total calorie intake, and if you are constantly over your TDEE each day, you are guaranteed to gain body fat. Diet sodas, on the other hand, don't have the calories or sugar, but contain many more additives,

chemicals and preservatives that are not easily digested by your body and throw off your entire internal functions, such as your endocrine system, which is responsible for your metabolism.

Also, carbonated drinks can give you a bloated or full feeling from all of the air gas contained in the drink. This can be uncomfortable and certainly inhibit your ability to stay active.

Am I saying to never have a soda again? Absolutely not, but do enjoy your favorite regular or diet soda only in moderation. My recommendation is to have no more then 3-4 soda drinks per week in order to maximize your results.

2. *Alcohol* – Bottom line is this: alcohol is toxic. It literally is a poison. I won't sit here and preach to you to never have a cocktail or a beer ever again; that is not reasonable. In fact, one of my favorite things in this world is a piece of dark chocolate with a glass of red wine. But, I need to explain to you the ramifications of drinking alcohol to your goal of burning fat and changing your life.

First, alcohol dehydrates you. That is why it is such a natural enemy of water. It does the exact opposite of what water does to your body. You now know what happens to your body's ability to burn fat when you are dehydrated. It doesn't have that ability! Your organs are too busy trying to get rid of this poison you have ingested.

Second, alcohol is a slow killer. The damage that excessive alcohol does to your body is insurmountable. Some effects of abusing alcohol include heart disease, stroke, liver disease, diabetes, high blood pressure and cancer, just to name a few.

Third, alcohol is high in calories. We know that protein and carbohydrates have 4 calories per gram, and fat has more than double of that with 9 calories per gram. Well, alcohol has a whopping 7 calories per gram, putting it a close second behind fat. That means the liquid calories you take in when you drink alcohol add up more quickly than soda or sugary drinks do, which can lead to fat gain and retention. Not to mention that most alcoholic beverages are full of "empty" calories with almost no nutritional value.

Finally, alcohol prevents your body from utilizing the nutrients of your food. The metabolizing of good protein, carbs and fats virtually shuts off when alcohol is present in the body. What does that mean for you? That means that your muscles can't build and stay strong from the protein you eat, you can't get any energy from the carbs you take in, and the fats are getting stored away immediately rather than being used to maintain good general health! Your body is too busy trying to figure out what to do with the alcohol in your system.

So what amount of alcohol is okay? As a guideline, I coach my clients to keep moderation with alcohol, which means 1-3 drinks per week for females and 2-5 drinks per week for males. And by "drink" I don't mean the 24oz. special draft beer at the bar down the street; I mean regularly portioned drinks. Enjoy a drink or two here and there, but if you are really serious about your goals and your progress, you will keep alcohol in strict moderation and treat yourself when you've earned it. As for the social aspect of drinking alcohol, anyone who truly cares about you will support your decision to use alcohol only for special occasions or in moderation.

3. *Sports Drinks* – Since the 1980s, sports drinks have gained popularity as a way to stay in the game and be your best athletically. They are heavily marketed as performance enhancers, endurance and strength maximizers and edge-providing wonder-drinks. Is all the hype really true?

My answer is two-fold. On one end, you've got your endurance athlete, the marathon runner, the long distance cyclist or the tri-athlete. For this person, maybe these drinks make sense. When you are highly active for more than one hour at a time, your body will need some easy replenishment of simple sugars and electrolytes, without feeling the need to stop and eat. In this case, a sports drink probably makes a lot of sense. So the question is: do you fall into that category?

I'm guessing no, as most of my clients, and myself included, are not long distance athletes. So, on the other end of the spectrum is us regulars. We are just folks that want to be lean, strong and healthy. We want to look and feel our best. In our world, sports drinks really offer no real benefit. The result is that we are drinking a flavored sugar water that will not only add liquid calories to our daily intake, but also will have sever effects on our blood sugar levels, causing us to release insulin and store body fat.

My best advice is to enjoy sports drinks in moderation, or stay away altogether if your number one goal is to lose body fat.

4. *Juices From Concentrate* – Many types of juices are sold in our grocery stores each day. The two basic types of juice you will find are (1) juice not from concentrate and (2) juice from concentrate. Juice that is "not from concentrate" generally means that the juice you are getting is just from the fruits and/or vegetables only, with nothing added or taken away. Of course, this isn't always the case, so you should always read the label to find out what is actually in the container. These types of juices are okay, but should be used only once in a while or in small portions because the liquid calories do add up.

The juices that are "from concentrate" generally have additives and other things added into the juice to either make it last longer on the shelf or taste enhanced. Oftentimes if you read the label of a juice from concentrate, it will tell you how much actual juice is contained. For instance, the label will say "Contains 5% juice." Much like diet sodas, those extra fillers and additives usually don't bode well for your internal systems since they are completely unnatural and have adverse effects on your health as well as your ability to burn fat.

If you must drink juice, again enjoy it in small portions every so often. Many natural juices do have healthy benefits. In order to get the best results out of your fat loss program, avoid any juices from concentrate whenever you can.

5. *Sodium* – Too much salt is not healthy for you regardless of whether or not you are trying to lose inches. A diet high in sodium can lead to high blood pressure, heart attack, kidney failure and even death! I'm sure that is

not news to you. Too much salt can also dehydrate you severely, as well as give you a bloated look and feeling.

When I coach my clients towards their goals, I teach them to never add salt to your food. Salt will find its own way onto your plate, especially if you eat out at all or have any kind of deli meats. If you must add salt, choose sea salt rather than table salt, and use it only in moderation.

Also, if you find yourself having a meal or a treat very high in sodium, be sure to compensate by drinking some extra water. Since salt retains water, drinking a little extra will help your body to flush out the excess salt and return your body to a proper water balance.

THE TRUTH ABOUT COFFEE AND FAT LOSS

I get inquiries about whether coffee is good or bad for you all the time, especially as it relates to your ability to burn fat. Coffee has its pros and cons, but altogether it is not a true enemy of water unless it is abused. The same goes for your ability to burn fat. Coffee only inhibits your fat burning progress if it is abused. Let me explain…

Here's the good news. Coffee comes from the Earth, it is a natural food choice provided to us by Mother Nature. In fact, a strong cup of coffee in the morning has actually been shown to give your body a metabolic boost and get your fat burning ability jumpstarted for the day. For many, coffee is seen as a ritual, maybe even something social that can bring people together for a conversation or comfort you on a cold morning. Many of my clients have shared with me that they simply cannot live without their cup of coffee, and I tell them, "You don't have to!" If you choose coffee beans that are pure and untampered with, I'm more than fine with that. In fact, I enjoy a cup of coffee to start *my* day. Highly processed or flavored coffees are less desirable, as they often have many fillers and unnatural substances that can affect your body's ability to function normally. Keep it natural.

However, here are a few things to keep in mind when considering your daily cup (or multiple cups!) of coffee. First, coffee is a diuretic, which means that it naturally flushes out much of your body's water, potentially having dehydrating capabilities. For that reason, do not overdo your coffee consumption. 1-2 cups per day should be sufficient, so be sure to enjoy it in moderation.

Second, it's generally what people *add* to their coffee that gets them in trouble trying to lose body fat. Heavy cream, whole milk, sugar, flavored syrups and even whipped cream are some everyday favorites for many people, and the calories and poor nutritional qualities of these choices leave people with nothing more than a few extra pounds of body fat each year. Drink coffee black or with as few additions as possible.

Lastly, it is not good to be addicted to anything, and caffeine can be very addicting. It is actually listed as a drug by the FDA. Monitor your consumption, and avoid becoming addicted to drinking coffee. This can lead to severe mood swings, migraine-like headaches and a large decrease in energy. None of these side effects are beneficial to losing body fat and getting healthy. Again, enjoy everything in moderation.

The bottom line with water and its enemies is this: stick to water as your main source of fluids. You cannot go wrong with water. Liquid calories add up quick and very rarely offer you much benefit when trying to lose body fat. Use coffee and natural juices in strict moderation; too much of anything isn't good.

RAPID RECAP

1. Water is your best friend. Not only will it keep you healthy, it is the most powerful way to burn body fat.

2. Our bodies are 70% water, as are our muscles. Without water, we cannot survive very long.

3. Be sure to have the proper amount of water based on how many calories you burn each day, and find what

works best for you.

4. Don't overdo water; cap it off at 12 quarts per day.

5. Beware of the enemies of water:

    a. Soda

    b. Alcohol

    c. Sports Drinks

    d. Juice From Concentrate

    e. Sodium (salt)

6. Enjoy coffee in moderation. It can actually help you in losing body fat. But don't overdo it and minimize what you add to your cup.

CHAPTER 8:

Supplement Myths and Truths: Do I need them to succeed?

"The doctor of the future will give no medicine, but instead will interest his patients in the care of the human frame, in diet, and in the cause and prevention of disease."
- Thomas Edison

The supplement industry is a multi-billion dollar industry. There are an estimated 100 new supplement products hitting the market each and every day! There are literally thousands of different companies out there trying to sell YOU their latest and greatest fat burning pill. We're talking big business here, and there does not seem to be any downward trend in the industry.

Want to know the scariest part of all this? The supplement industry is completely deregulated and free to advertise how they please and put whatever they want to in the bottle without fully disclosing its contents. That is downright scary!

Everywhere you turn, you find an advertisement or a commercial or even an article on how great a new product is at burning fat. The message is simple: "Eat whatever you like, don't exercise…just pop this pill and you'll be thin overnight! Guaranteed or your money back!!!" We have been brainwashed to believe these lies, and who can blame us? No hard work, no dieting, but all the results! Part of us desperately wants to believe this, so we do.

Does this mean that all supplements are bad and that any company trying to sell their product is evil? No, not at all. There are some good, reputable products out there. Because there are so many different choices and countless advertisements trying to win your business, it can be utterly confusing. I will clear up your confusion. Let's first address the different types of supplements, then I will explain everything you need to know about which ones to use and which ones to avoid.

TYPES OF SUPPLEMENTS

In an effort to keep this simple, there are only two basic types of supplements as they pertain to your fat loss program. The two types are (1) pills, powders and drinks, and (2) meal replacement products (MRP's). Virtually all of the weight loss supplements you will come in contact with will fall into one of these two categories. Let's take a look at each one and discover the truths and dispel the myths associated with these products.

PILLS, POWDERS AND DRINKS

The first type of supplement is all the pills, powders and drinks. More specifically as they pertain to this program, the *diet* pills, powders and drinks. Also, this category includes your vitamins, minerals and other pills, such as calcium or fiber pills.

This is going to be very brief and simple. Do not, under any circumstances, rely on any diet pills or drinks; they are gimmicks and they do not work. In fact, most of them are just plain unhealthy and potentially dangerous. You've all seen the late night infomercials or the ads in the magazines with the before and after photos. What a company might claim about a product is most often not true, and because of the deregulation of the supplement industry it is a virtual free-for-all when it comes to advertising. I cannot and will not recommend any fat loss pill on the market, period. If you choose to believe the lies and continue to have faith in fat loss gimmicks, then I'm afraid this program is not for you.

Fat loss pills are often called thermogenics for the thermic effect they claim to cause when you take them. In most cases, these products contain high levels of caffeine and other ingredients that do nothing more than get your heart pumping. There are obvious dangerous side effects that come with taking these pills and any reward that may come from taking them, real or placebo effect is not worth the risk.

No pill is magic, no drink will ever replace hard work, and your body is way too complex to ever be correctly and permanently affected by a nutritional supplement. Again, my advice: don't fall for it. Stay far away from any product that claims to increase your metabolism, burn calories without exercise or melt away fat without having to watch what you eat. I know that somewhere in your heart you know all of this is true. Stick with your gut feeling. You've been around this block once or twice, how many of these fad products with empty promises actually worked for you long term? Most likely none, otherwise you wouldn't need this program.

Now, the only pill or tablet that I can honestly recommend that would fall into this category would be a good multivitamin/mineral. The quality of our food and agriculture has deteriorated over time due to a loss in quality soil, pollution and the use of pesticides. As a result, our fruits, vegetables and other foods have lost a lot of their nutritional value. There are now gaps in the nutrition content of most off our foods, and we have to rely on multivitamin/mineral supplements to fill in those gaps.

Not all vitamins are created the same however. You should seek out a brand that is made up of vitamins and minerals from whole food sources with the least amount of fillers and additives. Your vitamins should mimic natural food as close as possible. Also, if you need to obtain fiber or any other nutrient that you are unable to get from food alone, by all means do so through food supplements. These supplements would also include folic acid, calcium, various additional vitamins, and iron, to name a few. These kinds of supplements are great for convenience and for general health, and you should inquire about their specific benefits to determine whether or not they are right for you.

MEAL REPLACEMENT PRODUCTS (MRP'S) – BARS AND SHAKES

The second type of supplement is the meal replacement products, or MRP's. MRP's are the shakes, bars and other products that attempt to take the place of a meal, usually including protein powder, carbs, vitamins and other ingredients. MRP's have three major benefits: (1) they offer convenience, since it is very hard to eat every three hours, especially if you are eating whole foods, (2) they can be cost effective and much less expensive than real food, and (3) they ensure that you will get enough protein throughout the day so you don't compromise your metabolically-charged muscle.

Are MRP's better than food? No, and they never will be. No matter what any company comes up with for a new MRP, at the end of the day it's just powderized food, nothing more. But, they certainly do have their place in a program like this, and I personally consider MRP's to be crucial to my own success. I simply don't have the time or desire to sit down and eat a whole meal every three hours. I'm sure you don't either. It's hard enough as it is! MRP's make it so much easier, whether it's a bar or a shake, because they are portable. I can plan my day and not have to worry about cooking food or making enough time to sit down and eat.

Just like anything else, MRP's are not all created equal. Some are really good, but most are not. Again, always read the label. When you are buying a bar or a shake mix for convenience, be sure to read what is in it. In this case, less is more. Go for the products that have less ingredients and minimal preservatives/additives. If you can't pronounce the ingredient list, don't buy it! Go for the more natural products. Believe me they are out there, you just need to look for them.

Also, when choosing an MRP that is right for you, be sure to choose a product that is well balanced with a good amount of protein, some complex carbs, low in sugar and saturated fat, and high in vitamins and nutrients. A solid meal replacement product should follow the 3:2:1 ratio of protein:carbs:fats. Read the label. It's all there.

IS THERE ANYTHING ELSE I NEED?

Are there any other products or supplements that you will need to lose body fat the correct and permanent way? Honestly? Nope. Stick to real wholesome food, and fill in the gaps with a good vitamin/mineral tablet and MRP's for convenience. Anything else you read about is probably a lie, even if the FDA backs it up. For years the only true recipe for losing body fat the right way is sound nutrition, consistent exercise and a healthy dose of discipline. This recipe has not changed over the decades, and it never will. Anything else is just a gimmick.

RAPID RECAP

1. The supplement industry is worth billions each year, and is totally deregulated.

2. Don't believe the hype. For the thousands of products on the market today, 99% are not healthy and do not help you lose body fat.

3. There are two types of supplements: (1) pills, powders and drinks, and (2) meal replacement products (MRP's).

4. Choose supplements to fill in gaps in your daily nutrition and for convenience only, not as an answer to your fat loss problems.

5. Seek products that are reputable and safe, and always read the labels!

SECTION III

THE ULTIMATE FAT BURNING EXERCISE PLAN (SIMPLIFIED)

CHAPTER 9:

Weight Training and Burning Fat

"Never eat more than you can lift."
- Miss Piggy

"I'm not into working out. My philosophy: No pain, no pain."
- Carol Leifer

Exercise is the last piece to your puzzle. There are two major types of exercise that are critical to your success: (1) weight training and (2) cardio training. Weight training is essential to reaching your fat loss goal, as is cardio training. You must have a balance of both in order to reach your personal pinnacle. In this chapter, I will enlighten you on the reasons why weight training is so crucial to burning fat and keeping it off, as well as provide you with some of the basics of weight training so that you can get started today. I will also clear up any confusion about weight training, because there are certainly plenty of myths concerning the effects of working with weights.

Now that we are on to the exercise portion of this program, it is important to take a pause and reflect on what I call the "Fat Loss Pie," and no, this is not the tasty kind of pie you may be thinking of. The Fat Loss Pie is a three-piece pie, consisting of three equal parts. The three parts of the pie are: (1) nutrition, (2) weight training and (3) cardio training. These three components are what make up this fat loss program, and each part is absolutely essential to your success.

The crust of the pie that surrounds these three parts is the first section of this book that focuses on goals and accountability. That "crust" wraps it all together, and if one or more pieces are missing, you are spinning your wheels. Every single one of my clients that has transformed their body took on some grueling weight training, grumbled through tons of cardio exercise, committed to a well balanced nutrition plan and wrapped it all up with a healthy dose of accountability and goal setting. You are no different. You are getting the same treatment. When these parts of the pie all come together, they create a synergistic result that leads to wellness, good health and aesthetic success.

WHY DO I NEED WEIGHT TRAINING FOR FAT BURNING?

Here are 3 major reasons why you MUST incorporate weight training into your routine if you plan on losing body fat and staying super lean:

1. *Muscle is metabolically charged* - If you haven't noticed yet, this program is all about one thing and one thing only: your metabolism. Muscle tissue is the most metabolic thing in your body. That means the stronger your muscles are, the more calories you will burn not only during exercise, but all throughout the day, even when you are at rest! Imagine burning more calories every day regardless of whether you are rested or active.

Without working out your muscles by doing some resistance training, your muscles start to wither away and they become weak. It's called the "Use It or Lose It," principle. You need to stretch and contract your muscles with added resistance in order to stay strong and metabolically charged. Otherwise, if you don't train your muscles, you will slow down your own metabolism and continue to store more body fat.

2. *Weight training prevents injury* – When you are strong, your body tends to put up with the daily wear and tear of living and staying busy. When you are strong, you tend

to be more flexible, with more range of motion about your joints, allowing you to take on your daily tasks with vigor, endurance and confidence. When you are weak, bad things happen. Your back goes out. Your knees ache. Your low back gets tight. You may even injure yourself. Believe me it happens every day to someone. When you are achy or even injured, your fat loss progress comes to a halt, and you are no good to yourself or anyone else for that matter.

Becoming and staying strong should be very high on your priority list. I have worked with many clients that were in their 70s and 80s that have not aged well at all, simply because they lacked the strength to let their body age gracefully. They made the choice when they were younger to ignore their bodies. Don't let that happen to you. Your results, and possibly your life and wellbeing, may depend on it.

3. *Weight training is an anti-aging activity* – Make no mistake about it, each day you are alive, you are slowly dying. Your metabolism is decreasing every year after you hit 30, and your muscles and internal organs eventually will deteriorate. Depressing, huh? Well, it doesn't have to be! You don't need to accept that! If you train with weights properly, together with a balanced nutrition plan and some cardio activity, you can reverse the aging process by keeping your metabolism high and your energy levels through the roof! Not to mention the health benefits from lifting weights, including a decrease in blood pressure, improved circulation, and lower cholesterol, just to name a few.

If you ignore this key activity, you will certainly face many health struggles as you age and you will "feel your age" if not worse. I cannot express to you in words just how critical weight training is to your health and your success at melting away stored body fat. Remember, it is 1/3 of the Fat Loss Pie.

COMMON MISCONCEPTIONS ABOUT WEIGHT LIFTING

There are many myths about weight lifting that I constantly get questioned on year after year. Most of you are confused, and I used to be too! But that ends now. Here are the top 7 weight training myths, and the real truth behind each one:

1. *I will get "bulky" if I lift weights* – I get this one from my female clients all day long. Sometimes I even get it from the men, too. Many of my clients were afraid they would "bulk up" simply by lifting weights, and I understand full well that a regular every day person, especially a female, does not want the bodybuilder look. That makes sense, and it's easy to see how one might be slightly afraid of what weight training can do to your body if you've ever seen some of the muscle bound athletes in a gym That's obviously not the look for everyone.

The bottom line is this: you will not get bulky from lifting weights, period. For all of the women out there who think otherwise, please allow me to explain. First of all, a woman's body is not designed to have large muscle mass. The hormones and muscle fiber types that are needed to grow muscle in freakish size simply are not present in the female body. All female bodybuilders are on steroids, which mimics a male's hormonal balance. Unless you plan on starting a steroid cycle, your body just won't accept the muscle gain. This is fact, not opinion. You can't change the way your body is made up physiologically.

Secondly, in order to gain substantial amounts of muscle mass one needs to eat an extremely high calorie diet coupled with extremely heavy weight lifting, neither of which are recommended in this program. It is very difficult to gain muscle size and mass, just ask any thin person who's tried to do it. Gaining significant amounts of muscle is hard enough to do consciously, let alone by mistake. Unless you plan on eating like a horse and training like a bodybuilder, I wouldn't worry about gaining too much bulk; it just won't happen.

The same thing goes for the men. This program is designed to help you lose body fat and look and feel your best, not gain excessive amounts of size and outlift everyone else in the gym. If your plan is different from this and you wish to do these things, then this principle won't apply to you. If you stick to this program, you will not bulk up.

2. *I don't need weights, cardio alone will burn the fat* – Cardio does burn fat. That is true. You will learn all about the benefits of cardio training in the next and final chapter. Many of my clients have argued that cardio alone has helped them lose weight in the past, and some even think that they need to lose the weight first with cardio then build muscle with weights. The biggest problem with this thinking is that your muscle is totally ignored, when your muscle should get the most attention. If your plan consists of just cardio, then the most metabolically active tissue in your body (your muscle) starts to fade away, causing a slowdown in your metabolism. When this happens, you might actually be losing weight. That's great, but it doesn't mean you are losing body fat. Much of the weight you lose on the scale could be muscle weight and water retention. The best approach is to have all three pieces of the Fat Loss Pie present: weight training, cardio training and nutrition. These three pieces will come together and create synergy in your lifestyle.

3. *I will get injured if I lift weights* – This concern can be real. I will freely admit that. Weight training can be abused and done very incorrectly, often times with serious ramifications. Injury may occur, both minor or serious, and you should always consult your doctor and a qualified fitness professional before beginning a weight training program.

However, if done correctly, weight training actually prevents future injuries and can help to rehab some old ailments by helping you gain strength and flexibility. Don't ever perform a movement that you don't understand, and never try to mimic what someone else does in the gym. Most people do not practice good form. So, while injury does and can happen, it should not be cause to not take on weight training, just make sure you approach it in the proper manner from the start. Seek out help if needed, and always err on the side of caution.

4. *Lifting weights turns fat into muscle* – Fat tissue and muscle tissue are two completely different types of tissue present in your body. They cannot turn into one another no matter how much body fat you lose and how much muscle you gain. How it works is this: your fat tissue covers your muscles. There are two types of fat on your body: (1) subcutaneous fat and (2) visceral fat. The subcutaneous fat is the fat tissue that lies beneath the skin, covering your muscles. The visceral fat is the internal fat that protects your organs. In regards to losing body fat, we are talking about both the subcutaneous and visceral fat, although the subcutaneous fat usually attributes to about 75% of your total body fat.

Again, fat can never be converted into muscle; it is physiologically impossible. Rather, what happens is this: as your fat cells shrink over time and you lose body fat, your muscles become more apparent and show better. Fat tissue is very spacious and it takes up a lot of room. Muscle tissue is very dense and lean, and does not take up much room at all. Also, muscle tissue weights approximately 4 times more than fat does, so as your muscle increases and your fat decreases, you become smaller but might actually weigh more on the scale! I know, it sounds crazy, and most of my clients freaked out when they saw the scale actually go up in the beginning, but let me reassure you, your body needs to change in many ways before you might see a drastic decrease on the scale. You might be gaining muscle weight in total, but losing body fat and inches. Judge your progress by taking circumference measurements and use your clothes as a true barometer rather than relying on just the scale.

5. *I don't belong in the weight room at my gym, only the muscleheads go in there* – Over the years, more and more people have realized the benefits of weight training for health and fat loss. As a result, the weight room at the local gym is not just for the muscle bound athletes

anymore. More and more everyday people are using the equipment during their workout, and generally most gyms these days are more than accommodating to anyone that might be a novice. You have every right to use that equipment in your gym, if you choose to work out in a gym setting. Your member fees are just the same as the next person. Do not let your own fears or assumptions get in the way of your progress.

The best advice I can give you is to find a place to work out that makes you feel comfortable, and once you join take advantage of the free training session most gyms offer new members. Once you start weight training and see some results, you'll be much more confident and you might even start to really enjoy your workouts.

6. *I will lose my flexibility by lifting weights* – I covered this a bit earlier, but a common myth about weight training is that it causes you to be muscle bound and to lose all of your flexibility. This could not be any more untrue! In fact, it's quite the opposite. Each and every time you perform a weight training repetition, you are stretching your muscle fibers, then contracting them, repeatedly until your set is done. Each rep has a stretch point, and your joints gain range of motion as you do this. Stretching has its benefits, too, but simply lifting weights correctly will increase your flexibility, not decrease it! The only surefire way to lose your flexibility is to decrease your activity. If you sit on the couch or at your desk all day without any movement or activity, your muscles and joints will certainly tighten up and lose flexibility. Weight training is never the culprit for this – being lazy is.

7. *I will do crunches every day to lose my gut* – How many times have you walked through a gym and saw dozens of people doing countless crunches and ab exercises in hopes of shrinking their waistline? It happens every day, and in fact most exercise gimmicks that are on the late-night infomercials involve some kind of crunch or sit-up motion.

Doing any form of exercise has tremendous benefits, so I would never discourage you from doing anything active. But, performing endless crunches in hopes that will solve your gut problem is something I need to clear up. Anytime you work your muscles, you are strengthening your muscles and in turn increasing your metabolism. You are NOT spot reducing and attacking the fat that is present in that area. Spot reducing does not work.

Small movements like crunches, bicep curls and calf raises all typically work just a single muscle and don't do much for fat loss. I'll discuss the best exercises to perform to lose body fat in just a bit. What you need to know is that by strengthening your entire body and revving up your metabolism, together with some cardio activity and proper nutrition, is what will get you the results you need for your entire body, the gut or any other trouble area included! Most of my clients never really had to focus on doing ab exercises because the exercises I included in their program indirectly worked their core enough without having to do crunches. I will share those exercises with you later in this chapter. Just remember, spot reducing doesn't work.

THE BEST WEIGHT TRAINING EXERCISES TO LOSE BODY FAT

So, what are the best weight training exercises that you can do to permanently lose body fat? There are literally thousands of different exercises out there, with just as many opinions and styles as to what is best. Over the years, many of the basic exercises have been expanded on and revamped, and new technology has enabled us to create totally new exercise platforms that challenge people of all fitness levels in completely new ways. Exercise really is a cutting-edge industry.

For me to go into each style and breakdown all of the exercises that you can choose from is simply impossible. I would have to have a completely separate manual just on this chapter alone, and this program is not designed for that purpose. Most of what you have learned thus far focuses on nutrition, since that is the one piece of the pie that can trump the other pieces. So, the most effective way to teach you the basics of weight training is to do just that – keep it basic. Despite all of the advances in training and techniques, the same exercises will always remain as your foundation for fat loss and strength.

Here is my all-time, most effective exercise list to help you burn fat, stoke your metabolic furnace and keep the fat off for life! I have split the exercise list into two major groups: () upper body and (2) lower body. If you stick to this list and make small variations and changes when necessary, you will see and feel the amazing fat burning results! These are the same basic exercises I use with my own clients as well as myself:

<u>Upper Body</u>

Bench Press

Military Press

Lat Pulldown

Chin Ups & Pull Ups

Dips

Chest Flyes

Lateral Raises

Front Raises

Dumbbell Rows

Barbell Rows

Upright Rows

Close Grip Bench Press

Pullovers

Curls

Shrugs

<u>Lower Body</u>

Squats

Deadlifts

Romanian Deadlifts

Lunges

Leg Press

Hack Squat

Leg Curls

That's it folks; pretty short list, huh? Some of those exercises may sound foreign to you, and that's okay. You can link up with a trainer for a session or two to learn these basics, or do some research online to find out how to do them. Again, this is not an exercise manual. There are just way too many variations on each of these movements to go into detail here. Take this list of basic but effective weight training exercises and get going on the next step…do them! You will burn fat and feel young, that I can guarantee!

THE DETAILS - REPS, SETS INTENSITY & FREQUENCY

Now you have the basics on why weight training is critical to your success, you no longer are confused about the myths of weight training, and you now have the list of the best fat burning exercises to get you to your goal. Now what?

Now you need the details of an effective fat loss weight training regimen. Those details include such things as how many reps and sets you should do, the proper intensity level and how much weight to use and the frequency of how often you should be weight training. My recommendations are not set in stone, I can only tell you what has worked for my clients in helping them transform their bodies. There are millions of possible combinations of reps, sets, etc. Here is the same routine I have used with hundreds of clients through the years.

REPETITIONS & SETS

A repetition is defined as performing one full range of motion for a given movement, counted as one. So, if you pick up a dumbbell and curl it up to your shoulder, then lower it down so that your arm is straight, that is one repetition, or rep. Several repetitions repeated over and over again for a given number comprise what is called a set. So, if you curl that dumbbell 10 times and stop, you've just done one set of 10 repetitions.

The optimal number of reps and sets for fat burning varies for each person, and the best thing for you to do is to experiment to find what gives you the best results. However, as a starting point as well as a surefire way to get results, this program teaches the following guidelines:

- 3-5 exercises per workout
- 2-4 sets per exercise
- 8-12 repetitions per set

This combination of exercises, sets and reps seems to work wonders at building lean muscle tissue, increasing the metabolism, burning fat and increasing strength. Some people see great results from higher reps and some from low rep counts. Is there a definitive answer? No, only what I have seen work time and time again.

WEIGHT TRAINING SPLIT ROUTINES

Your body is made up of many muscle groups, including your deltoids, pectorals, hamstrings, quadriceps and trapezius and latissimus dorsi, to name a few. Some of those you may know, some you may not. That is not important right now. The important thing to know is that you should split up the muscle groups that you workout into what is known as "split routines." This means that on certain training days you only work certain muscle groups. If you are a beginner, training your entire body for all three weight lifting days is just fine, since the intensity and volume of your workouts will be on the lighter side. As you progress, splitting up the muscle groups will be very beneficial so that you can focus on one or two muscles each workout and then give those muscles adequate rest until the following week.

For instance, a common three day split I use with my clients is:

Day 1 – Upper body push muscles (chest, shoulders, triceps)

Day 2 – Lower body (quadriceps, hamstrings, calves)

Day 3 – Upper body pull muscles (back, traps, biceps)

This split usually will contain rest days in between, and each muscle group is getting worked once per week. As training time increases and result ensue, the splits can become more complex to fit your needs.

TRAINING INTENSITY & FREQUENCY

Should you train to muscle failure? Should it hurt? Does "No pain, no gain" still apply? Should you train 7 days a week? How much weight is the right amount of weight? How will I know if I am lifting too much or too little? These are all great questions. The answers to these questions are critical to your success at burning body fat, and must be taken seriously.

First is the issue of training to muscle failure, or intensity. This means that you are performing a set of a given exercise, and you are unable to properly finish the last repetition without having your muscles totally exhaust and give out. Many fitness professionals believe in training to failure all the time, without exception. This is believed to be beneficial because it forces your body out of its comfort zone, thus forcing your muscles to react to this major change in what you body is used to. This is called the Progressive Overload principle, created by one of fitness's legends, Joe Weider.

Progressive overload is a great principle to follow because it implies that you are constantly improving your performance week after week and pushing yourself. However, in your world, pushing to muscle failure does not have to be achieved all of the time. First, it can be very dangerous, and you should only push to failure if you are training with a partner or have a spotter. Second, unless you are an advanced weight lifter, your muscles will not be ready for the shock of training to failure and you could injure yourself very easily. In order to simplify the question of intensity, I use a 1-4 scale with all of my clients in order to properly measure the intensity of a set.

1 –too light, can perform over 15 reps and more with little or no effort

2 –moderate weight, proper form, muscles close to failure at last rep but could manage 2-3 additional

3 –heavy, maintained good form, last rep was final rep with proper from, maybe could achieve 1-2 more

4 –too heavy, lost form, reached failure before optimum rep range of 8-12

This simple intensity scale should be applied after each set you do, and let your answer guide you toward your next set. If you are at a 1, increase the weight until you find the proper amount. 2's and 3's are ideal, and if you reach a 4, decrease the weight. You should never dread your workout because you are too sore to walk; that is not productive. Your body should have a comfortable yet deep soreness so that you know you trained hard but not over the edge. Keep in mind that this intensity scale uses what's called a "perceived rate of exertion," which basically means that a 4 to you could be a 1 to me, and you must use your own best judgment when assigning a number to your completed set. All that matters is how the set feels to you.

Next comes the speed of your repetitions. Depending on your goals, you can vary the speed at which you perform an exercise. Every weight training movement you do will have two phases, a stretch and a contraction. For purposes of this program, the ideal rep speed should be 2-3 seconds during the concentric phase (lifting the weight and contracting the muscle) and 2-3 seconds during the eccentric phase (lowering the weight and stretching the muscle).

This speed allows for the perfect amount of muscle reaction that causes a metabolic increase.

Then you must consider the rest time in between your sets. Once you finish a set of 8-12 repetitions you will need some kind of rest to charge up your muscles again and prepare for the next set. My training philosophy has always been to rest minimally in between sets, keeping your rest time to 45 seconds or less. I often use supersets with my clients as well, which is two consecutive exercises back to back without any rest. This accomplishes two things: (1) it minimizes your rest time, keeping your heart rate up causing you to burn more calories, and (2) makes your workout that much more time efficient.

As for weight training frequency, I recommend 3-5 days depending on your fitness level. If you are a beginner, start with three days of weight training. If you are advanced, up to five might be the best volume for you. There really isn't any need for more than five, no matter what level you are on. The bottom line is your body needs rest. You don't actually get stronger when you lift weights. You get stronger when you rest *after* lifting weights. When your body heals itself from the workout, your muscles heal and increase in strength, thus increasing your metabolism. If you don't ever rest, you become catabolic, or in a state of muscle wasting.

Also remember to switch things up every so often. Your body has a natural adaptive ability to change when it is faced with prolonged physical stress caused by weight training. This is called the Adaptation Syndrome, which states that your body will get used to any routine if you keep it constant for long enough. If you keep the same weight training regimen for too long, your body will stop reacting in a positive way. For this reason, you must shake things up approximately every 4-6 weeks. Ways to do this include changing the amount of weight you lift, the order of your exercises or even the speed at which you perform your sets.

Finally, your weight training workouts should not last any longer than one hour. In fact, 30 minutes is ideal for strength training. I say this for two specific reasons: (1) after the one hour mark, your body starts to use your muscle as a source of fuel, because the carbs in your system have been depleted and a combination of stored fat and muscle mass become the fuel source. This is not good. I'm sure you've picked up on the theme of this program: never sacrifice your muscle; it's what drives your metabolism. (2) If your workouts are much more than one hour, you will start to feel a time burden and most likely quit. Most of us do not have the time or desire to spend more than one hour working out. For endurance athletes it's a different ballgame, but for people that want to lose fat and look and feel their best, stick to this guideline.

RECOVERY FACTORS YOU NEED TO SUCCEED

There are five critical recovery factors you need to properly heal from your weight training workouts and get the results you need. They are (1) protein, (2) water, (3) sleep at night, (4) rest days between workouts and (5) stretching.

The important thing to know is that you do not get stronger when you weight train. What you are doing to your muscles during training is called "micro-tearing" the fibers and you are actually causing little mini-injuries to the tissue. That is why you get sore after a workout or any other activity your body is not used to. After your workout is done, your muscles need to heal in order to recover and grow stronger, thus leading you to a higher metabolic rate and further fat burning. In order to heal properly, you need all five of the recovery factors to be present and on point. Otherwise, your muscles will quit on you and become catabolic. Let's learn more about each recovery factor and why they are so critical to your success.

1. *Protein* – As discussed earlier, protein is the building block for your muscles. Your muscles are made up of protein and water. Without adequate protein after your workout and throughout the day, you simply cannot keep your muscle mass. You fall into what is known as a "negative nitrogen balance" and your muscles eat away at themselves to get the protein you're not giving them!

2. *Water* – Water is so critical we dedicated a whole chapter to this one recovery factor earlier in the program. When you are dehydrated, your muscles are dehydrated. When that happens, your muscles shut down, your body shuts down, and you are no longer burning fat. In fact, you begin storing fat as a survival mechanism. Water is your best friend. Don't neglect it.

3. *Sleep at night* – I'm sure you've heard that an optimal night's sleep is a full 8-10 hours. Well, you heard that for a reason. Not only is that amount of uninterrupted sleep good for your health, it is also critical for your fat loss success. When you are not fully rested, your body releases stress hormones that cause you to gain and retain body fat. Also, your workouts cannot be performed at peak performance, so you lose on that end as well. Get some sleep, and make sure it is seamless through the night for 8-10 hours.

4. *Rest days between workouts* – You cannot train with weights every day. You need to learn that your rest days are the days that you are improving your body. You train hard, you rest hard. If you overtrain, and believe me there is such a thing, your body will shut down quicker than you can imagine. Do not fall into this trap. Plan your rest days, ideally in between your workouts. For instance, work out on Mondays, Wednesdays and Fridays, and rest on the other days in between.

5. *Stretching* – Flexibility is key to your success because it helps you in your training routine as well as prevents injury. When you have a decent amount of flexibility about your joints and muscles, you can perform your weight training exercises with better form and increased safety. Also, stretching after your workouts will increase blood flow to your muscles and help them to heal. Always stretch *after* exercise and rarely before, as stretching a cold muscle can lead to injury and a loss in strength. Be sure to be warmed up and/or finished with your routine before stretching.

6. Maximize the amount of recovery factors you practice each week and you will exponentially increase your results. Without these five factors of recovery, your fat loss progress will be slowed down.

RAPID RECAP

1. There are various reasons why you must weight train to properly lose body fat. The most important reason is that muscle is the most metabolically active tissue in your body. Never sacrifice your muscle for anything.

2. Don't believe the common misconceptions about weight training; it really is safe and acts as an anti-aging process!

3. Keep your routine simple, and master the basics of weight lifting first. Use the guidelines of reps, sets, intensity and frequency to maximize your fat loss.

4. You must recover from your workouts in order to lose body fat. If you don't recover properly, your body will not react positively to your workouts.

CHAPTER 10:

Cardio Training and Burning Fat

"Few people know how to take a walk. The qualifications are endurance, plain clothes, old shoes, an eye for nature, good humor, vast curiosity, good speech, good silence and nothing too much."
- Ralph Waldo Emerson

"Jogging is very beneficial. It's good for your legs and your feet. It's also very good for the ground. It makes it feel needed."
- Charles M. Schultz

Cardio is the last and final piece to this program. I know, some of you may be cringing at even reading the word "cardio," but it is necessary. As a matter of fact, cardio training is the one activity that will burn the most fat for you. Remember that in order to lose body fat you must bring your body into a calorie deficit. You can choose to eat less, which is what most of us have done in the past. You now know that causes the starvation response and is not an effective long-term plan. Or you can choose to eat more and burn off the excess body fat. Cardio, together with weight training, is the activity you need to do just that. You will need cardio to succeed just like you will need a well balanced nutrition plan and some weight training. Remember the Fat Loss Pie.

The definition of cardio as it pertains to this program is "any aerobic activity that elevates your heart rate and keeps it elevated for an extended period of time, preferably 20-60 minutes in duration." The word "aerobic simply means "with air," and assumes that the activity you are doing involves oxygen flowing through your bloodstream, which happens when your heart rate is elevated for an extended period of time.

This chapter will explain the reasons that cardio training is critical to you success, as well as identify and clear up any myths or confusion you may have about cardio. Lastly, it will provide you with you a simplified cardio plan so that you can start burning away fat immediately.

WHY DO I NEED CARDIO?

There are three basic reasons why you absolutely need cardio training as a crucial part of your fat loss program. Here they are:

1. *Cardio burns a lot of calories* – when it comes to burning calories, cardio is tops! Any cardio activity is going to burn more calories for you than any weight training routine you can muster up. In order to bring your body into a calorie deficit, you need to burn calories! Cardio does that for you. It is virtually impossible to be in a calorie deficit without cardio activity for a period of time without invoking the starvation response. So, by incorporating cardio into your weekly routine, you are burning the stored fat calories rather than trying to starve them off. If done properly, cardio can burn an extra 200-1,000+ calories per workout. That adds up to some serious fat loss if done multiple times per week.

2. *Cardio burns fat* – one of the main sources of fuel for your body during cardio is your stored body fat. Not only does cardio push your body into a calories deficit, it actually burns the fat on your body as its fuel source! We'll talk about fuel sources in just a bit, but it is important for you to know that your stored body fat is like premium fuel for a cardio workout.

3. *Cardio is integral for maintaining and improving your health* – not only will cardio help you to look your best by melting

away body fat pounds, it will also get you healthy! Health benefits from cardiovascular exercise include lower blood pressure, lower cholesterol, improved circulation, less stress, improved endurance, lower risk of stroke or heart attack and increased energy among many others. The list goes on and on. Aerobics can give you health, increase your health or even maintain your health.

COMMON MISCONCEPTIONS ABOUT CARDIO TRAINING

1. *I don't need cardio, diet alone will do just fine* – If you diet, you will likely lose weight. Of course, that weight loss will most likely be water weight and muscle loss, due to a severe prolonged calorie restriction. Then, when you fall off the wagon, your body will balloon back up because you've wreaked havoc on your metabolism. It is for this reason alone that this program exists. I tell you to eat! I tell you to burn your body fat, don't try to starve it off! As a result, if you are eating the proper amount of calories per day to maintain good health and promote a high metabolism, then you must burn off the excess fat with activity – that activity comes in the form of weight training and cardio training.

Cardio is where you will actually burn the most calories *during* the activity you are doing. With weight training, you're burning calories *after* the workout because resistance training supports an increase in your metabolism. You simply need both forms of activity in order to keep your metabolism high and burn enough calories to force your body into a healthy deficit through activity, not through starvation.

Make no mistake about it, if you skip cardio, you are shorting yourself the results you need and want. You can't lose body fat effectively and permanently without raising your heart rate through movement and burning extra calories. Period.

2. *I have to do hours and hours of cardio to get the real benefit* – this is completely false. Oftentimes people will make the assumption that in order to get great results they have to spend countless hours on the treadmill or the Stairmaster. I am telling you that is a lie! If you are an endurance athlete, then maybe long distance cardio sessions is what you need to perform at your best. But for the everyday person looking to shed body fat and be healthy, your cardio sessions can be anywhere from as little as 20 minutes up to no more than 60 minutes to accomplish your goals. I will talk about the different options of time spent on cardio in just a bit. For now, the point I am making is that cardio does not have to be viewed as a chore or as a severe time commitment. Too many of my clients in the past and present have told me that they skip cardio because they feel if they can't do one full hour than why bother? There are many ways to not only make cardio fun and interesting but also to make it time efficient.

3. *Cardio is boring!* – Well, I guess this can be true for some people. I will admit I don't love cardio all that much. In fact, I downright hate it! But, it is necessary, and oftentimes the best fix for this problem is to try new things and never do the same routine twice. Perhaps if you go into a cardio session thinking it's going to be boring, guess what happens? It becomes boring. 95% of your success depends on your attitude, and that holds true for your workouts.

A great tool I use with my clients is to tell them to remind themselves that they will be leaner and more fit when they are done with their workout than when they began just a few minutes ago. Imagine the fat just melting away and burning off the more you keep at it! Use music as a motivator. Play your favorite songs during cardio, typically faster paced tunes that will get you going. These are just a few examples of how to get through the cardio doldrums.

4. *I can't run, so why bother at all* – walking is the best activity you can do for your body, bar none! There is no better or more natural way of moving your body than walking, and

> virtually anyone that is able can do it! It's free, it requires no equipment and you can move at your own pace! You can even wander to new places or appreciate nature at its finest. Many people feel that because they are out of shape or even can't run due to ailments they can't get the wonderful benefits of cardio exercise. That is bunk!

Any form of cardio that you can handle is better than sitting on the couch! Walking, cycling, jogging, skating, swimming, hiking, dancing, running and playing sports all are great ways to get your heart rate up and burn calories, you don't need to be a marathoner to do this! So many people I have worked with would consider themselves to be "all or nothing" type of personalities, which can be dangerous when it comes to working out. Don't be hard on yourself, do what you can and do your best. Any amount is better than nothing.

THE BEST FAT BURNING CARDIO PROGRAM EVER! (AND ANYONE CAN DO IT!)

There are thousands of theories that exist on which form of cardio is best for losing body fat. Is high intensity or low intensity cardio better? Should I do intervals or steady state cardio? Should it last hours or just minutes? When should I do my cardio? Before or after weight training? The list goes on and on. What follows are the best fat burning guidelines I can give you on the ins and outs of what you need to do to maximize your fat loss using cardio training as a key component of your program. The best part of this cardio program is that anyone can follow it because it applies to both fitness beginners and advanced athletes alike. It will be customized to you. There are several parts to this piece of the pie, so let's begin.

DETERMINING YOUR TARGET HEART RATE

Before you begin any kind of cardio program, it is important to calculate your Target Heart Rate (THR). I always use the Karvonen

Method of calculating heart rate targets, since it is the most accurate and it factors in your resting heart rate as a place to start. This way the calculation is highly customized to each client. The Karvonen formula is a simple formula that calculates the optimal heart rate for burning fat and improving cardio health. Here are the steps to calculating your cardio target heart rate.

First, you must test your Resting Heart Rate (RHR). This is defined as the number of heart beats you have in one whole minute while at rest or as close to it as possible. The ideal time for taking this measurement is when you wake in the morning. Simply check your pulse on your neck or at your wrist and count the beats while you time yourself for one entire minute. The average number of heart beats in one minute for a healthy adult is around 72 beats. If your heart rate is much higher then 72, then you may have a low cardiovascular threshold. If your number is much lower than 72, you may have a much better cardiovascular threshold and be in good to great shape. Medications and/or pacemakers may also play a factor here. I often use the resting heart rate as a general gauge to someone's cardio fitness level.

Next, you must calculate your Maximum Heart Rate (MHR), which is basically the maximum number of beats per minute your heart can handle when put under severe physical stress. This part is simple. Just take the number 220 less your age. So, if you are 40, your MHR is 220 – 40 = 180bpm, or beats per minute.

Then you can calculate what is called your Heart Rate Reserve (HRR). You do this by subtracting your RHR from your MHR. Let's say for example that you are 40, and your resting heart rate is 72 bpm. Your HRR would be:

220 – 40 = 180 (MHR) – 72 (RHR) = 108bpm (HRR)

Your HRR is 108bpm, which is saying that you have 108 beats per minute on reserve for you to use when exercising.

Next, you would apply your HRR to whatever level of cardio intensity you feel is accurate for your fitness level. The ranges for intensity are as follows:

65%- beginner level w/ light/medium cardio exercise

75% - moderate level w/ somewhat intense cardio exercise

85% - advanced level w/ high intensity cardio exercise

So, building on our example, if you are at a moderate level of fitness, then your calculation would be:

108 X .75 = 81bpm

Finally you would take this number and add back in your resting heart rate to get you target heart rate of 81 + 72 = 153bpm.

Now you have your target heart rate for your cardio workouts. This is a great place to begin safely and it will let you know the optimal heart rate for burning fat. Keep in mind that this calculation is merely a guideline and is not 100% accurate. You will never consistently hit your target heart rate all of the time, so use a range. I use a range of +/- 15 bpm's with my clients. You will learn more about the types of cardio and how they affect your heart rate in just a bit, but you must use your own gut instinct on what feels right for intensity. For some people, their heart rates can soar very close to their estimated maximum heart rate with no problem, and others seem to always have a very low rate. Use good judgment.

TIMING IS EVERYTHING!

With cardio exercise, timing is crucial. While there is no right or wrong as to when to do your cardio training, there are significantly better times to maximize fat loss. The most important factor to consider when determining the best time to get some cardio work done is your body's source of fuel for your cardio. Let's discuss the different fuel sources when doing cardio, and then we'll nail down the best times to do it.

Your body has three fuel sources it uses for energy to perform an activity. These three sources of fuel are called "metabolic engines," and they include phosphagen, glycogen and oxygen. These three engines are what allow your body to perform any movement you can imagine, and depending on the speed and duration of that movement, your body calls on one of these fuels to get through the activity.

The first fuel source that your body calls on when exercising is phosphagen. This is a natural fuel source manufactured in your body for very brief, intense movements, generally lasting no longer than 10 seconds in duration. An example of this type of exercise would be a very short but fast sprint.

The second fuel, or metabolic engine, is glycogen. This is basically carbohydrate stores in your bloodstream that provide you with the energy needed for exercise that is moderate in length, generally lasting from 10 seconds to several minutes in length. When you weight train or do aerobics after having eaten during the day, your body uses glycogen to get you through the workout.

The last metabolic engine is oxygen, or air. As stated above, the word aerobics means "with air," meaning that oxygen is present when you perform long duration exercise. Your body uses oxygen as its source of fuel when your exercise lasts in excess of several minutes and continues to go on.

It is important to know about the three different sources of fuel for exercise because you can manipulate your workouts to call on certain sources of fuel to benefit your fat loss progress. For instance, your body burns stored fat when oxygen is present in your bloodstream, so long duration exercise is most beneficial for burning fat. You want to be exercising with the oxygen metabolic engine in order to tap into your stored body fat. Also, it is critical to know that when you have glycogen stores in your system and you keep your cardio duration moderate, then your body will need to burn the glycogen before it taps into the stored body fat.

So, with that information known, there are some ideal times to perform your cardio workouts in order to maximize your fat burning. Firstly, doing your cardio first thing in the morning while fasted is ideal for fat loss. This technique, called "fasted cardio," takes advantage of the fact that your body has been resting all night and is fasted, so any activity done at this time will burn fat instead of having to burn any glycogen, or carbs, in your system. Your body knows that you haven't eaten yet and therefore have no fuel to get moving, so it calls on your stored body fat as fuel. This is a very powerful way to stimulate fat loss, and should be considered if you are serious about your progress.

Secondly, if you cannot do this (or wish not to do this), there is another way to simulate this technique. If you combine your weight training routine with some cardio as well, ALWAYS perform your cardio workout AFTER doing your weight lifting. While weight lifting, your body will use glycogen as its major source of fuel, burning up virtually all of the carbs you have stored as fuel. Once that is done, and you begin your cardio, you will be in a fasted state, much like you would be when you wake in the morning. You are in effect performing fasted cardio.

Lastly, with these two scenarios aside, there is no wrong time to do your cardio. Any activity will help to push your body into a calorie deficit, so don't be too strict on the timing, just do it. That's the bottom line: get it done any way you can, and focus on timing only if your lifestyle permits.

HOW LONG SHOULD MY CARDIO SESSION LAST?

There are many theories on what the best duration of cardio is for burning fat. Some enthusiasts claim that long duration is the only way to truly burn fat, while others swear by short, intense cardio sessions. So which is it? The best answer is both.

Long duration, or "steady state" cardio, is widely known as a great fat burner. Steady state cardio gets its name from the increased yet steady heart rate pace that one keeps while performing a long distance cardio session, such as jogging or cycling. Once your heart rate is up, it stays up and maintains a high level, causing your body to use the oxygen engine as fuel and burns fat as a result.

Remember, when oxygen is present, fat is burned. This happens when your cardio session is anywhere from 10 minutes in duration or longer, and in the case of this program, no longer than one hour. Remember, after one hour your body may start eating away muscle mass, which is the last thing you want if your goal is to burn fat and look your best.

Your goal is to raise your heart rate to your target heart rate, which we calculated before, and keep it there for as much of you cardio session as possible. Keep in mind your target heart rate is just a guideline; you will know if you are in the proper fat burning zone by giving yourself the "conversation test." This works by asking yourself the following question while completing your cardio session: "Am I working hard so that I feel tired, but still can hold a conversation with someone next to me?" The answer to this should be "yes." If you are gasping for air and unable to sustain your pace, you are working too hard. If you can hold a conversation but feel that you could last at your current pace for hours, you are not working hard enough. Find a happy medium, and be honest with yourself. This will lead to unbelievable success for fat loss. I have seen this work for myself as well as countless clients that I have helped transform. I can honestly say that steady state long duration cardio is great for burning fat.

On the other hand, very short yet intense cardio sessions have a tremendous effect on burning fat as well. These types of aerobic workouts call on the phosphagen and glycogen metabolic engines to provide your body with fuel, and generally involve some kind of interval scheme. Interval schemes are quite the opposite from steady state cardio, in that an interval scheme is when you have a period of very intense output followed by a recovery period, repeated over and over again.

For example, a typical interval scheme would be running very fast for one entire minute followed by walking for one minute to recover and prepare to repeat. These workouts are typically anywhere from 10-30 minutes in length, and should be much harder than your steady state workouts.

The benefits of this type of cardio are twofold. The first benefit is that you will usually burn a higher number of calories during a shorter period of time with interval training, leading to an even bigger calorie deficit for your day. A bigger deficit means more fat loss.

The second benefit is that your metabolic structure changes when your body is forced out of its comfort zone. When your body performs at a very high level of intensity, your metabolism shifts upward and must react to the changing environment and conditions that you are forcing on yourself. Interval training lends itself very well to a high metabolism. This is because your body knows to adapt to the same routine when it is performed many times over. Intervals help to shake up your routine and introduce a new training regimen to your body.

Always remember that intervals and shorter, more intense cardio workouts are not for someone that is just starting a workout routine. You must work your way up to using this strategy. Please note that when using high intensity interval training your heart rate may be elevated even higher than your target heart rate and then quickly decreased during your recovery periods. This is not for the faint of heart (no pun intended!). However, also keep in mind that interval training does not subscribe to the theory of being in the "fat burning" heart rate zone; it focuses more so on high intensity work that pushes your body way out of its comfort zone.

It does work, though, very well in fact. I can vouch for interval training as a way to shed fat pounds. A great example of this type of training is competitive sprinters. Have you ever seen an overweight sprinter? You probably haven't, because they don't exist. All sprinters do is high intensity interval training since most sprints only last 10-20 seconds in length. Sprinters tend to have a very low body fat percentage as a result of this type of cardio training. Clearly, using intervals as part of your program is a powerful way to reach your goals and burn fat as well.

There are three basic interval programs that I use with my clients that cater to the three different metabolic engines of your body, which are again phosphagen, glycogen and oxygen. These interval schemes have been created and are endorsed by CrossFit, a leading authority in advanced training and wellness. The programs are as follows:

Metabolic Engine	Interval Scheme (high:low)
Phosphagen	1:3 ratio (30 seconds high: 90 seconds low)
Glycogen	1:2 ratio (1 minute high: 2 minutes low)
Oxygen (fat)	1:1 ratio (2 minutes high: 2 minutes low)

These three basic schemes follow a certain workload ratio that provides you with a guideline for balancing your high speed and low speed durations. You can alter and change these to fit your abilities and goals, and there are infinite possibilities of combinations when doing interval training. I tend to utilize the oxygen 1:1 ratio with my clients because they can get the benefit of interval training while using their oxidative engine, which promotes fat loss, since oxygen is present.

The point is this: both steady state and interval cardio should be used to get the best results in burning fat. Don't swear by one or the other, because both techniques and durations will give you fantastic results! Switch things up often. That will keep the results coming in as well as keep your routine fresh and fun.

THE RIGHT INTENSITY FOR YOU

So what's the right cardio intensity for you? There is no one answer for everyone, since we are all different people with unlike fitness abilities and goals. The old school thought was that your fat burning "zone" was approximately 50%-60% of your target heart rate, which is a very low intensity level. This theory is actually posted on many cardio treadmills and elliptical machines in popular gyms as a guideline for you. This theory claims that the majority of the proportion of calories that you burn at this level of intensity will actually be mostly from stored fat, so it ignores total calories burned but focuses on the type of calories burned. While there is some truth to this theory, you will see much better results if you focus more on the total number of calories burned during your cardio workout rather than where those calories come from.

For instance, if you walk on a treadmill for 45 minutes and keep your heart rate in the 50%-60% range of your target heart rate, you may only burn 150 calories. Those calories could very well be all stored fat calories, but the number is much lower than if you pushed to a higher intensity. The best scenario is to burn as many calories as you can so that you will be in a greater calorie deficit by burning calories rather than starving off calories. For that reason alone, high intensity is preferred over low intensity.

As a rule, you must only do what your body can handle. If you are just starting out, low intensity very well could be the only option for you, and that's okay! Just do it, don't worry about the intensity just yet. But as your fitness level increases and you start to see and feel the results, you then have a choice to start pushing harder. The only two ways to create a larger calorie deficit in this program are: (1) push harder and longer during your workouts, and/or (2) workout more often during the week. Find the right combination for you and your situation.

When writing cardio programs, I always use the 1-4 scale of perceived exertion with my clients when measuring the intensity of cardio workouts. Here is that scale again:

1-Too easy and light, can push much harder, recreational cardio

2–Moderate cardio intensity, burning significant amount of calories, some room for increase in difficulty

3–Very High intensity, perfect balance of pushing hard but not overdoing pace and heart rate, high calories burned

4-Too difficult, losing breath, unable to recover, not sustainable for entire duration

The goal is to obtain some 2's, and lots of 3's. Minimize the 4's you encounter, this level of cardio is not effective or safe. Always use your best judgment, and make sure that at the end of the day you are progressing rather than regressing.

FREQUENCY OF CARDIO WORKOUTS

Lastly, how often should you do cardio? Some fitness professionals will tell you to do cardio every day. Some will tell you that you don't need cardio to lose body fat. That's two separate ends of the spectrum, so whom should you believe?

In theory, your body is designed to perform some kind of cardio movement every day of your life. When humans were hunters and gatherers, we had to venture out and find our food each day. That included walking, running and swimming on a daily basis while we hunted. We have evolved since then, and today most of us know where our next meal is coming from. As a result, the amount of activity in our daily lives has decreased tremendously. But our bodies can handle movement if we decide to include it in our daily routine. Cardio is different than weight lifting in this regard, since rest days from using weights are critical to your success at losing body fat. You don't need too much recovery and rest from cardio exercise, aside from extremely long-distance aerobics.

Does that mean that you need to do cardio every day of the week? No, not necessarily. You could, and if you choose to do that you will certainly see great results. Most of us are very busy with work, family obligations, personal commitments, etc. and daily cardio might not be reality. Nor might you desire to do daily cardio! My official recommendation for cardio frequency is a minimum of three days per week and a maximum of daily cardio, or seven days per week for optimum fat loss. Most of my clients that have seen great results make it a weekly commitment of 3-5 cardio sessions per week. Of course, there is no right or wrong. The obvious answer is to only do as much cardio as you need to achieve your goals.

RAPID RECAP

1. Cardio is a must if you want to lose body fat correctly and maintain good health.

2. Cardio is the one activity that will burn enough calories

to bring your body into a calorie deficit each day.

3. You should determine your target heart rate to use as a guide during your cardio workouts. This will keep you safe and allow you to measure how you are doing.

4. The best times to do cardio are first thing in the morning while you are fasted, or after weight training, or any time. Just do it!

5. The frequency, intensity and duration of your cardio sessions are up to you, just do your best. 3-5 days per week for no more than one hour is a baseline point to get started. You should cycle in high intensity interval training with some moderate intensity steady state cardio to maximize your fat loss results.

CONCLUSION

(This is just the beginning...)

Congratulations! You've made it to the end of this program, and I sincerely hope the information was presented to you in simple terms and that you fully understand what you must do now. I have given you all that you need to succeed. I also hope that you are able to take this information and share it with your friends, family and even your children. By now you have mastered the following principles of losing body fat:

- You know why all diets die and why we are in trouble as a society. Knowing the problem is half the battle; taking action to fix it is the other half.
- You have crystal clear goals that will act as your new roadmap to success.
- You learned all about accountability and you must now obtain an unbiased accountability source.
- You are a master at the basics of nutrition. You know the concrete laws of losing body fat, as well as the fundamentals of the three macronutrients, as well as the critical role of water.
- No more gimmicks for you; you are too smart to fall for the infomercials, the supplement ads and the fad diets. You know what supplements you should use and which ones to avoid.
- You are armed with all you need to get started on a weight training and cardio training exercise regimen, which will help you to burn off stored fat rather than trying to starve it off.

The next step is all on you. Your road ahead will not be easy by any means. You've come this far by investing your time to read and retain the information in this program – don't stop now! I sincerely wish you great luck and success in your quest for health. Trust me – you can do this!

I believe in you, just like I believed in the thousands before you who have taken this journey. Make your change a lifestyle change and not a quick fix. Your results from here on in are permanent. Commit to that.

In an effort to help and coach you along, I am making myself available to you through email. You can reach me at my personal email address, jpantera@alldietsdie.com, anytime you wish to chat. I would love to hear about your success as well as push you along if you need my help. How's that for accountability? If you have questions, comments, struggles or victories, I am here for you.

Now, get going! You've got a lot of work to do and there is no better time than right now!

Sincerely,

John L. Pantera, CFT SPN

www.ingramcontent.com/pod-product-compliance
Lightning Source LLC
Chambersburg PA
CBHW020239290526
45784CB00003B/1034

9781438981864